Contents

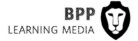

Contents

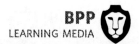

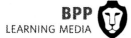

Contents

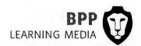

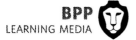

About the Publisher

BPP Learning Media is dedicated to supporting aspiring professionals with top quality learning material. BPP Learning Media's commitment to success is shown by our record of quality, innovation and market leadership in paper-based and e-learning materials. BPP Learning Media's study materials are written by professionally-qualified specialists who know from personal experience the importance of top quality materials for success.

Free Companion Material

Readers can access a free bonus chapter, 'The Limping Child', online.

To access the above companion material please visit www.bbp.com/freehealthresources

About the Author

Edward Snelson MBChB MRCPCH DRCOG DCH

After working as a GP partner for five years, Edward decided to become a hospital paediatrician based on a desire to spend all of his time doing what he enjoys most, treating children. He is also an enthusiastic teacher of colleagues and medical students. During his career, Edward has gained a great deal of experience treating children and teaching in a variety of environments. It is with this in mind that he has written this book as a quick reference guide to help doctors deal effectively with common paediatric problems.

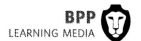

Acknowledgements

Although there are too many people to list who have contributed to my love of paediatrics and writing, it is easy to know who to thank first. My amazing wife Maria, and my superb children Daniel, Naomi and Theodore, are unquestionably the only people for whom I can say that if it were not for them I would never have written this book. Their support, encouragement and wisdom have truly been the reason why an idea has become a textbook.

I can now only apologise for the fact that I cannot name all of the people who I have worked with over the past couple of decades who have been teachers, mentors, colleagues, and students. I should also thank each child and parent that I have tended to, since experience is the best teacher. Every encounter, discussion and collaboration (including any moments of panic at four o'clock in the morning) have helped me to come to a point where I think I can make a degree of sense on the subject of how to assess and treat children and their many illnesses. Some of those people who have contributed the most know who they are, but many don't, and it is of course genuinely true that the greatest progress up the learning curve occurs when you make your greatest mistakes. I thank the children, parents and colleagues who were there at those times doubly.

Finally I would like to thank, in no particular order: Emily McArdle, Greg Brown, Lindsay Lewis, Emily Jamieson, Elizabeth Toberty, Laura Drabble, Sarah Green, Alison Liddle and Alan Gibson who read through my initial ramblings, gave me feedback and helped to turn a 'brain dump' into a manuscript. I hope that you are all pleased with the final result. Thank you also to all the people at BPP, especially Matt Green and Ruth D'Rozario, who have guided and encouraged me in this project.

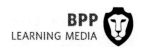

Foreword

Kids can be scary!

This isn't an admission of being bewildered by contemporary youth culture. I mean that paediatrics can be a daunting specialty. I know only too well that having to deal with a sick child can make a doctor's heart – especially if the doctor is young or inexperienced – beat faster than almost any other clinical situation.

With a young patient, the stakes often feel higher than with an adult. Young lives seem somehow more precious, more vulnerable, more dependent on the doctor getting it right. When the patient is a child, the consultation becomes a much more complex process. It usually involves dealing with parents, whose worries and expectations, understandable though they are, put the doctor under more pressure. Clinically, too, assessing an ill child can be particularly challenging. The history often has to be obtained from a third party. The child's response to being examined is unpredictable. Things happen fast; a child can look right as ninepence one minute and be practically moribund the next. Spotting 'red flags' is more important than ever. Every doctor's list of nightmare scenarios includes a screaming infant, panicking parents, deteriorating clinical signs and everyone yelling, '*Do* something!'

Wouldn't it be nice to be able to take such situations in your stride, confident that your knowledge, clinical acumen and interpersonal skills were equal to at least most of the paediatric problems you as 'doctor of first contact' are likely to encounter? Of course it would. So read Edward Snelson's excellent book.

The primary care of children doesn't just take place in general practice. If you work in an A&E department, or a Paediatric Assessment Unit; if you work as a locum or for an out of hours service; or even if you work in a quite different specialty but have friends who ask you about their children 'rather than bother the doctor', your self-esteem and your reputation will surely benefit if you can tell a sick child from a well one and can manage common paediatric problems competently.

Edward Snelson is the ideal author for this purpose. Already an experienced GP, he went back into hospital paediatrics because he loved treating children so much. The reverse journey – from hospital-based to community practice – is not unusual. Sadly, doctors who make it are not always very good at managing common conditions or handling the clinical uncertainties that general practice is full of. But I'll wager that Edward Snelson's hospital colleagues (and his patients) have gained a lot from the practical wisdom, the empathy and the good way with words with which his time as a family doctor has equipped him.

A reassuring '*You can do this!*' message pervades this book. All the common and important clinical problems are covered, as well as more tricky ones such as the child with 'funny turns' or possible non-accidental injury. The sections are organised by presenting symptom, and, as you would expect, each covers key points in the assessment and up-to-date management, including the things you must and must not do. What you might *not* have expected (but will be very grateful

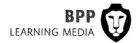

for) is advice about how a paediatrician in secondary care might deal with your patient if you have to make a referral, and also some useful suggestions about how to explain what's going on to parents.

Let me tell you a secret. Quite a while after I had agreed to provide this Foreword, Edward Snelson phoned me to apologise for the manuscript being so long in coming: 'NICE *will* keep updating their guidelines,' he explained, then added, 'I do wish they wouldn't!' I'm sure this seditious thought occurs, increasingly frequently, to every doctor. But medicine never keeps still, and the last word on any part of it will never be written. In the meantime, the best we can do is the best we can do. Much of what we think we know is probably sound, but quite a lot of it is doubtful and other parts are downright wrong – and, the trouble is, we can't always tell *which* parts. So we have to know what to do when nobody really knows what to do. That's what being professional means. Faced with this everyday paradox, we have only well-informed common sense to rely on. Edward Snelson possesses well-informed common sense in spades, and his book is infectious. Reading it, you yourself will catch a dose not only of his common sense but also of his delight in front-line paediatrics. Maybe kids aren't so scary after all.

Roger Neighbour

MA MB BChir DSc FRCP FRACGP FRCGP
Former general practitioner, Hertfordshire
Past President, Royal College of General Practitioners

Introduction

The first thing to realise is that **Paediatrics is a lot of fun**! (You will notice that the most important learning points are in bold throughout the book, the first one is probably the most important of them all.) I stopped being a GP after 5 years as a partner not because I was fed up with general practice, but because I loved being a doctor to children. Paediatrics is fun, because children are fun. You can blow raspberries at them and get paid for the time spent doing so. Paediatrics is also rewarding because it is very much how medicine used to be. Do you remember what you imagined yourself doing when you decided to be a doctor? Was lowering the nation's cholesterol a major incentive for you to become a doctor? Well, the great news is that most of paediatrics still involves treating (wait for it....) illness. What's more, the patients almost always get better.

So if you are going to be the top of the class in any branch of medicine then paediatrics is the one to be confident in. It's good old fashioned medicine, and there really isn't that much to it. Really, it is quite easy. There are just a few tricks to the trade, which are easy to remember, so read on.

I will provide an outline of how to approach a variety of common paediatric problems, starting at the beginning of life and moving though childhood. If you look at all the life-threatening conditions that children are prone to, it becomes a wonder that any of them survive. Fortunately they seem to be able to withstand these trials well. Our job is to decide which children would benefit from our marvellous medicines, and avoid medicalising the remainder. There is a tendency in paediatrics to overdo things because of our natural anxiety for children's wellbeing. I would never discourage anyone from agonising over every sick child. However, it is equally good for child and parent alike to avoid unnecessary tests and admissions to hospital.

Finally, before you read on, I would like to point out that I have not forgotten how little time you have in the general practice (GP) surgery or the emergency department (ED) to assess problems and make decisions. The guidelines I have written are as detailed as I can make them without making them cumbersome, but hopefully simple enough to use once you feel that you have a good understanding of the problem. By spending a little extra time with these problems when they present, I believe that you will avoid unnecessary investigations, ensure that you identify genuine problems earlier, and generally feel more satisfied with managing these conditions. I have written this book with the hope that you can use it both as a textbook at your leisure and as a quick reference book when under fire. For this reason there is a combination of detailed explanations and quick reference lists and flowcharts. So may these pages help you to enjoy practising medicine, and to show your paediatric colleagues that they don't really have a monopoly on being a know-it-all.

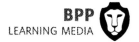

How to get the most out of this book

> Every effort has been made to ensure the accuracy of the material contained within this guide. However it must be noted that medical treatments, drug dosages/formulations, equipment, procedures and best practice are currently evolving within the field of medicine.
>
> Readers are therefore advised always to check the most up-to-date information relating to:
>
> - The applicable drug manufacturer's product information and data sheets relating to recommended dose/formulation, administration and contraindications.
> - The latest applicable local and national guidelines.
> - The latest applicable local and national codes of conduct and safety protocols.
>
> It is the responsibility of the practitioner, based on their own knowledge and expertise, to diagnose, treat and ensure the safety and best interests of the patient are maintained.

The aim of this book is to provide you, the clinician, with a guide to children who present with common clinical scenarios, and to managing the most common and important childhood conditions. In order to allow you to get as little or as much information, whenever it suits you, I have divided each chapter into sections. You may be reading this book at your leisure, in which case you are likely to read through each chapter in full. However, when you need it the most, you may have limited time to consult text, so I have organised each chapter to provide a brief guide and important points at the beginning. Although the chapter as a whole is still relevant and useful, for those in a real hurry there is a quick reference guide to each condition to help you when you have mere seconds.

The '**background**' should put each condition in context, and ensure that you understand the principles behind the assessment of each condition. This is not intended to be a comprehensive textbook so you will be disappointed if you are looking for chemical pathways and lots of statistics. Most paediatric textbooks are rich with rare syndromes. Instead, this book is intended to provide what the textbooks usually don't: a descriptive approach to clinical problems. If you are preparing for exams, then this book may need a companion and I would recommend that you also use a text which explores all of the facts that will be asked in examinations. I have avoided overburdening myself or the reader with too many figures. However for those sitting exams and learning statistics, facts and figures are a necessary evil.

The '**how to assess**' section tells you what to look for. Use this to ensure that you are assessing the most important signs and symptoms. If you have limited time, you may wish to read this and then look to the quick reference guide.

The '**must do**' and '**pitfalls**' sections are there to help you to provide best care for your patient and at the same time avoid disaster. In many ways these sections represent the opposite of evidence

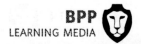

based medicine. This section is based on my successes and failures as well as the experiences of all those with whom I have worked. The recommendations that you find here are based mainly on the following categories of evidence:

- I do this and it works.
- When I don't do this it all goes horribly wrong.
- A colleague whom I respect told me to do this and it has always worked for me.

The '**management of**' section and flowchart provide one possible approach to managing the given scenario. This is not intended to be a comprehensive guideline, but rather an outline of how to keep the management within the boundaries of common sense medicine. You may also have departmental or practice guidelines and though I hope that mine will not differ widely, you should defer to your local guidelines. There are also various national guidelines for many conditions. NICE (National Institute for Clinical Excellence), SIGN (Scottish Intercollegiate Guidelines Network), and many of the colleges and societies have produced guidelines, some of which are good and simple to follow, and some of which are complicated and controversial. Remember two things when you are confused by guidelines:

- Firstly, a guideline is not a protocol. Ultimately you must use a guideline as a decision-making tool, but you have both the right and the responsibility to make decisions based on all the information that you have and apply this to the patient in front of you.
- Secondly, when multiple guidelines exist and conflict, there is probably no one right answer. The important thing is to make a management decision and be able to justify it. Sometimes the best decision is 'I cannot manage!' in which there is no shame.

The '**how to be a know-it-all**' section is part fun and part serious. If there was anything vital to consider I would have included it in the above sections. However while doing a good job in medicine is satisfying, it can be quite rewarding to be 'that doctor who's a bit good at...' I believe that if you only ever work at the level where you do the job well enough (and so manage to deliver care to more patients, which is also good) then you are at risk of becoming fed up, bored or even burnt out. One way to combat this is with occasional feelings of smugness. When you are the person who first considers a rarer cause for something, or spots a reason to consider another diagnosis, then you may be the person who picks up the reason why the patient isn't getting better. So in order to help you with this I have tried to include a couple of 'what if's for each chapter. Beware though, the features of rare syndromes are often the same as the common conditions. It is easy to start seeing zebras when really you are most likely to be encountering horses. Whatever you do, retain your sense of proportion and remember that common conditions are indeed common. However, if you have the time and don't abandon your common sense, you may find yourself enjoying a smug feeling as you receive startled admiration for your depth of paediatric knowledge. The '**also worth knowing**' bits are simply there as further information. I hope that they add understanding as well as trivia.

The '**role of the paediatrician**' section is aimed at those of you who are referring patients to secondary care. I believe that it is useful to know what happens next in order to understand when to refer and to give parents and children some idea of what might happen next, but please never use the words 'I am referring you to hospital for these tests.' This causes great distress

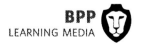

for doctors and parents alike when expectations are not met. I prefer to tell people that 'I am referring you to a colleague who may wish to do some tests'.

The **'FAQs'** section are there to answer specific questions that often arise when considering how to manage the condition in question. If I am ever asked the same question twice, I will add it to this section.

Finally, the **'what do I tell the parents?'** section is just that – it is what *I* tell parents. Parents are hanging on your every word when you give them the summary of your assessment and management plan. Their child is very precious to them, and parents have a tendency to imagine the worst case scenario. For this reason, I tend not to shy from both honesty and optimism when I explain the situation. Of course, we should not be blunt and we should not make false promises such as 'everything will be fine' when a child is ill. You can always say 'this condition can be serious, but I am very hopeful that your child will respond well to treatment' without being misleading or unnecessarily pessimistic. It is important to avoid the use of jargon and confuse parents with complicated explanations. Keep explanations simple and check that you have been understood.

So please use this book firstly to make sense of what really matters in assessing common childhood illnesses. If it helps you to pass an exam, then all the better! However, medical knowledge and clinical practice are partners who need to be introduced to each other, and I hope that this book will help to you to do that.

Note

'Parents' and 'carers' are used interchangeably throughout this handbook to refer to anyone who is taking care of a child.

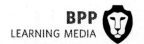

A guide to assessing any child who presents to general practice or the emergency department

Paediatric assessments are different to taking a history from and examining an adult. In its essence, assessing a child is a simple process. The clinician evaluates the history, forming an idea of possible diagnoses. There is then some form of examination which may rule out or confirm a diagnosis. Finally a decision is made whether or not to do further tests, to treat or to reassure and whether or not a referral is needed. Although the process is similar to assessing adults, the way to do this effectively is different and **an age-appropriate approach must always be used to reach a sensible assessment.** Use the following principles to help you to get as good a picture as possible of the child in front of you.

Approach each consultation with flexibility and inventiveness

Because children come in all shapes and sizes and each situation is different, adaptability is the key to getting the maximum amount of useful information. Examinations in particular are likely to be worked around the child. Take your chances while you can! If a baby is asleep, examine them early on, and be careful not to wake them. If a toddler shows a willingness to be examined, do so straight away because they may change their mind in a moment.

Talk to the parent and the child

Unless the child is pre-verbal, it is always worth engaging with the child. Although for most children the history will come predominantly from the responsible adult, talking to the child helps to establish rapport and allay any fears that the child may have. The older the child is, the more actual history that they can contribute. By teenage years the history should be coming primarily from the child, though it is still important to establish what the parent's concerns and agenda are.

Take a good history

Because most children have had a relatively short and uncomplicated life (so far), you are unlikely to get as bogged down with past medical histories or drug histories as you would with an older person. This leaves more time to concentrate on some other aspects of the history that may be more relevant and informative. Because time is precious and histories need to be focused however, it is important to know which bits are useful and when.

- **Birth history.** This is useful information mainly when dealing with a newborn or if the problem has any developmental aspect to it.

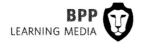

- **Feeding.** This is useful in most histories. For babies it is crucial to find out what, how much and how often the child is consuming. For older children, any information about recent changes in eating habits is probably more useful.
- **Immunisations.** Asking about vaccinations will give you an idea of the likelihood that the child may have any particular infection. It also sometimes gives you cause for concern when a child is unimmunised. Finally if there have been missed vaccinations you now have an opportunity to address that.
- **Family history.** Because there is less past history to give clues in children as to what illnesses they may develop, family history is very useful. As well as asking about conditions that the parents and siblings have or have had, the other sibling can give clues as to what is 'normal' within that family. Are they all short, or all tall, for example?
- **Development.** Check if they are reaching their milestones. Chronic illness can affect development. Developmental delay can also be a clue to underlying neuro-developmental problems.

Look at the child

More than in any other specialty, in paediatrics your assessment will be guided by your gut feel for each child you see. Although you cannot rely entirely on your first impression without taking a history and examining the patient, I would say that your impression of the child as a whole is as important a part of the assessment process as either the whole history, or the entire detailed examination. This is because it is possible to have a similar history from two children, one of whom looks well and the other who seems unwell. If you see a child with a history of a cough and who has crackles on examination yet runs up and down the corridor pretending to be an aeroplane, you can almost guarantee that they do not have pneumonia. However if you find nothing specific in the history or examination yet you ignore your gut feeling that something is not right about the child (even if you cannot put your finger on why) then you will fail to identify seriously ill children.

Airway, Breathing and Circulation (ABC)

If a child looks unwell then this should be your mantra for the assessment process. Although ABC is usually associated with the order of priority in a resuscitation, the aim in children is to treat illness long before they become ill enough to require resuscitation. You should therefore satisfy yourself that each (airway, breathing and circulation) in turn is adequate; if problems are found in any of these three areas you need to act in a way which will address that problem as soon as possible.

It is generally accepted that in the context of life threatening conditions, airway problems are more dangerous than breathing problems. In turn breathing problems are worse than circulation problems. This is because when an airway obstructs, it usually does so suddenly and the immediate result is severe hypoxia. **If an airway is partly obstructed enough to cause a noise then it may be about to get worse and this can occur with devastating speed.**

In turn a breathing problem will cause a child to succumb more quickly than a circulation problem. The other reason for assessing and treating problems in this order is that there is no point having a circulation which has no oxygen to deliver.

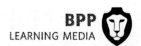

Make the examination fun

Going to the doctor can be frightening. Also, children are rarely motivated to cooperate just because you want them to. After all, you are a stranger and the child is unlikely to see any benefit from being examined. Furthermore, while some parents will try to persuade their child, many will see it as your responsibility to achieve a physical examination and will be quite passive.

The way to win this little challenge is to **make the examination process fun**. I find that a purposeful yet playful approach works best. In other words, I tell the child what I am going to do in a playful way but I follow through and examine the child unless completely impractical. This way the child knows that I am playful but also in charge. If the child realises that they are in charge then they will be more likely to refuse. A battle with the child must be avoided, so time spent enrolling the support of the parent and getting the child's co-operation is time well spent.

It is crucial to remember to **use appropriate language**. If you say 'I need to examine your ears' to a six year old you are unlikely to find that this is met with willingness to be examined. After all, what does 'examine' mean to a child of that age and what are you planning to do with that pointy thing? No thanks. However if, for example, you say that you have a light that helps you choose which medicine will make them better and tell them that it might tickle, you have a greater chance of co-operation.

Try these other approaches as well:
- **Get down to the child's level**. It is often necessary to examine a child while they play on the floor. Try to make sure that you don't tower over them.
- **Approach the examination in stages**. Try a friendly request and gauge the response that you get. Then show an interest in what the child is doing. If you go straight in waving your stethoscope without giving the child a chance to appraise you and the situation, you will most likely have a battle on your hands.
- **Preschool children are almost universally proud of the size of their abdomen but completely unaware that they even have something called a chest.** I suspect that this is to do with food. The bit between your mouth and your stomach seems to be an irrelevancy to all children of this age. So when I want to examine a chest or abdomen, I ask them, 'do you have a big tummy?' and 'can you show it to me?'
- **Children have a very good sense for people's moods and attitudes.** The more that you enjoy yourself with children the more they will tend to relax and cooperate.
- **Never use the word 'hurt.'** People usually use this word in the context of 'this won't hurt' or 'I promise not to hurt you', but the child just hears the word 'hurt' or imagines that you wouldn't mention 'hurt' unless it was a possibility. Instead, use a positive euphemism such as 'I want to feel your tickly tummy. You can tell me to stop if you need me to.'
- **Finally, bribery and blackmail are entirely reasonable tactics to resort to.** Sweets and stickers are usually welcomed and occasionally successful, although always try to get the parents permission to avoid upsetting them for example by giving the child something which they are not allowed.

Take the parents (or carers) seriously
Parents will usually know more about their child and what has been happening than anyone else. If you listen to what they say then you will find out much more than if you do too much of the talking. As mentioned later neither can you take all that is said at face value. Often parents will

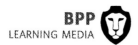

make statements which need interpreting and clarifying, but dismissing parental information and concerns is a recipe for disaster.

Indeed, parental anxiety alone is a recognised indication for requesting a further assessment. If you have not reassured the parents that their child is well, then I would advise asking yourself the following:

- Am I confident in addressing the parent's concerns? (If not then consider asking a colleague who works with you to review the child before referring or sending the child home.)
- Have I directly asked the parents/carers what their concerns are?
- Have I answered all their concerns and questions?
- Have I explained the condition and why I am happy with the baby?
- Have I made sure that the parents understand what to do if something changes?

If you have addressed these issues then you should consider referring the persistently anxious parents. There may be issues that they cannot or will not articulate to you. It is also worth being aware that these referrals sometimes bring other issues to the attention of the paediatricians, such as mothers with severe postnatal depression, the only clue being the carer's apparent unreasonable anxiety.

Examine what you need to

If you adopt a systematic approach and examine all children using a standardised routine you will be successful only some of the time. Children are often only intermittently cooperative if at all. Therefore use what knowledge you have of the problem which you are assessing so that you can prioritise your examination.

While a paediatrician would more often aim to fully examine the child (albeit in any order possible), GPs and emergency medicine doctors must learn to strike a balance between doing too brief and too thorough an examination. For example, it will be appropriate to omit a full neurological examination on most children. It is rare however to imagine not examining the chest, heart, abdomen and ears/throat of an unwell child. Aim to do as thorough an examination as time and the child will allow.

Risk-taking and safety-netting

Every clinical decision that you make involves a certain amount of risk. If you do not take risks then you are not practising good medicine. The bulk of children who come to be assessed acutely every day have viral illnesses which respond only to symptomatic treatment and the passage of time. Treating all of these children with antibiotics is poor practice, as is over-referring or admitting too many children. Instead we have to rely on a thorough history and examination, an appropriate clinical decision and good safety-netting.

Safety-netting is the process of equipping patients and carers with an understanding that illnesses change and that any plan made at the time of consultation may need to be reviewed if circumstances require it. It is inevitable that if you see enough children in your career, you will

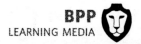

see a child who has an apparent minor illness and who later develops a life threatening illness. Some people respond to that by always giving antibiotics or referring or admitting too many times. However this is unnecessary and potentially harmful. If a child later becomes severely unwell then parents are likely to be reproachful only if they felt that their child was inadequately examined or they were poorly informed.

My approach is to err towards not treating or referring but to share as much information and risk with the patient or carer as possible. Be seen to examine the child thoroughly. Explain what you think is wrong with the child and what has formed that conclusion. Advise them about specific circumstances which should trigger the seeking of a further assessment (eg a non-blanching rash). Finally empower them to trust their own judgement. Sometimes children re-attend too late because the carers are assuming that the original assessment still applies despite quite marked deterioration and partly because they are worried that they will be seen as anxious if they consult twice for the same problem. For this reason **never tell parents that 'it is only a... (virus etc)'**, and always tell them that a minor illness only makes a child moderately unwell, so if the child seems worryingly ill, a secondary problem may have developed. **Parents must be reassured that if their instinct tells them that their child is not ok, they will not be criticised for seeking a re-assessment.**

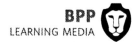

A guide to the terminology used to describe ill children

I have given explanations of some of the most difficult aspects of the examination to put into words. All of these are assessments that we make without always fully understanding them. I hope that by unpacking these you will find it easier to make a more confident assessment of these things which are an essential part of assessing any child.

Altered consciousness

Note that altered consciousness and drowsiness are terms that crop up in many places in this book, as it will do in any guide to managing acute paediatric conditions. It is usually a sign that something is severely wrong, most commonly hypoxia, dehydration or sepsis (especially meningitis). However important it is to identify altered consciousness, it is also sensible to avoid disturbing a sleeping child if you can manage to examine them without causing upset. So, since children spend so much of their time sleeping, especially when mildly unwell, how can you be satisfied about the state of their consciousness?

The answer is that the altered consciousness of illness looks and is quite different to sleep. **If a child has sepsis, or hypoxia or a head injury severe enough to depress cerebral function, they will be very unwell** and they will not look as they would if they were just sleeping peacefully. If you want to be sure, gently check their tone. I believe therefore that it is reasonable to document that the child was asleep, but looked well and had no signs of hypoxia, cardiovascular collapse or meningism. If you need to wake the child, that is of course also fine.

Assessing whether a child is systemically unwell or well

One of the best indicators of how well a child is comes from observing or enquiring about what they do. Children are much more straightforward than adults and as a rule do not have a desire to show a doctor how poorly they are. Illness is a serious inconvenience to children. As a result most children who come to a general practice or the emergency department see new toys and new people, and set to work straight away, exploring this new environment. It is this tendency which causes parents to lament about how very unwell their child was at home and how they feel that the little darling has made a fool of them. I find it reassuring therefore to see a child doing what they want to do, whether that means a baby feeding, a toddler running away to explore a corridor or a teenager sitting and arguing with their parent. **A child who does what they normally do is very unlikely to be dangerously unwell.**

In this context, I believe that some of the best information that can be obtained about a child from an examination point of view is actually gathered while a history is taken. While the history is being taken from a parent or carer, the focus is at least physically away from the child. During this time they may or may not be listening, but their behaviour is more likely to reflect their true state than when you come to examine them. Many children become like different people as soon

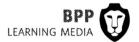

as you turn the attention to them. Since behaviour is one of the most important things to assess in examining a child, take note of how the child is before you examine them. If necessary, after you have examined them, you can take the spotlight off them again and regard their behaviour at this point as more true to how they are feeling.

Another good discriminatory finding comes from the history. Many children present with a history that makes the child sound more unwell than they seem at the time of assessment. Some of this may be due to parental anxiety. More often, the parents acknowledge how well the child looks. In these cases the child probably was much more ill and has now improved. Children's illnesses often follow a course of fluctuating symptoms. In my experience, this is a reassuring sign and makes serious infection less likely than if there is a progressive deterioration.

Respiratory distress

Assessing the signs of respiratory distress requires only that you remember your physiology. The point of respiration is to obtain oxygen and remove carbon dioxide. The lungs do this primarily for the benefit of the brain. When this process is failing there are various coping strategies which the body employs. These compensatory mechanisms or the failure of these mechanisms to work are what you are looking for. In practice, you are looking for two main things: the work of breathing and the efficacy of breathing.

Work of breathing increases as soon as a child's ventilation is compromised. This is the way that the body compensates for something which is adversely affecting respiration. Increased work of breathing can be an indicator of an airway problem or a breathing problem and is sometimes due to a circulatory problem. The signs of increased work of breathing are:

- An increased respiratory rate
- Use of accessory muscles – in older children this is noticeable by their position and by seeing the shoulder and neck muscles tense. In babies the use of accessory muscles may be apparent by the presence of 'head bobbing', a phenomenon where the head moves towards the chest with each inspiration.
- Tracheal tug, intercostal recession and subcostal recession
- Grunting – in order to stop their airways from collapsing, children sometimes grunt involuntarily when they have respiratory distress.
- Nasal flaring – in newborns this may be the only sign along with raised respiratory rate.
- Difficulty speaking (or crying)

These are all signs that a child is trying harder to obtain oxygen and/or remove carbon dioxide. They will usually manage to do this with great efficiency for a considerable amount of time. As a result, children can have signs of respiratory distress and remain remarkably cheerful. However, this is only sustainable for so long and should not be taken for granted. **Respiratory distress should be considered an early warning sign that eventually, the child may deteriorate and potentially do so rapidly.**

Efficacy of breathing is the term used to describe whether the child is no longer managing to maintain physiological levels of oxygen or carbon dioxide. The indicators of reduced efficacy of breathing are:

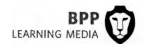

- Drowsiness, agitation or potentially any sign of altered consciousness
- Reduced tone and general floppiness
- Cyanosis and low oxygen saturation
- Reduced respiratory rate
- Compensatory tachycardia and then eventually bradycardia
- These children look very unwell
- Pallor (blood is being diverted to oxygenate the brain and heart)

These are all signs that compensatory mechanisms have now failed. It is very important to understand that **when a child shows signs of reduced efficacy of breathing, this is a sign of impending disaster.** Unless immediate action is taken, the child is at serious risk of death.

Assessing vital signs

Normal values for vital signs in children change greatly as they grow up. Each child is different and it should always be remembered that a single measurement is a snapshot of these signs. However since in an initial assessment a snapshot is often all we have, you need to have some idea of what is normal for an age group. The figures below are a guide to help you in your clinical decision-making, however it is nonsense to say that there is such a thing as a true normal range since it is not just age but weight and other contexts which determine what a child's vital signs should be.

Age	0–1 year	1–5 years	5–12 years	12–18 years
Resting heart rate	100–150	80–130	70–110	60–100
Respiratory rate	30–45	20–35	15–25	12–20

Note that quoted normal values for vital signs vary greatly and cannot apply to all situations (for example crying, pain or anxiety). The above figures are relatively generous and to be used as a guide; they are only useful if the signs are taken in context. However, it is important to note vital signs because they are almost always abnormal in the presence of serious illness. **You should therefore only dismiss abnormal vital signs if you are convinced of the wellbeing of the child.**

Another parameter which is useful in assessing acutely unwell children is capillary refill time. If done properly this sign is a useful part of the overall assessment. To measure this, gently press with a fingertip over the skin on the child's sternum for five seconds. Then measure the time that it takes for the blanched skin to return to the same colour as the skin around it. **The capillary refill time should be less than two seconds at all ages.** Note however that cold skin will give a prolonged capillary refill time. Capillary refill time is often misleading in the cold, febrile or crying child.

Prolonged capillary refill time, if assessed properly and centrally, indicates that there is probably a significant compromise to the circulation. This sign should be used along with heart rate and the overall appearance of the child to help determine whether there is a problem with the child's perfusion.

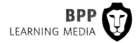

Chapter 1
Neonatal jaundice

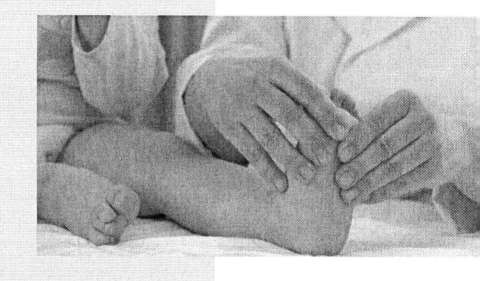

Neonatal jaundice

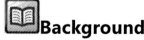

Background

The jaundiced baby can be a real quandary for the doctor when the child presents. We know that most babies with jaundice are well and get better on their own. However we are also aware that too much bilirubin is bad for you. Doctors may find that they deal with neonatal jaundice infrequently because the vast majority of these babies are observed by midwives.

Neonatal physiology makes jaundice all but inevitable. Besides a high rate of red cell breakdown, and an immature liver, there is the relatively poor fluid intake of the first few days. All these factors conspire to make babies develop jaundice.

Most babies who develop jaundice have physiological or 'breast milk' jaundice. A few will have a serious and dangerous underlying reason for their jaundice.

Some of those with physiological jaundice will have it mildly, while some will require treatment. It is not necessary to do blood tests in all cases, however it is vital to never allow jaundice to reach the point where it can do harm. Knowing when to act involves a quick and simple assessment in the first instance. This will allow you to determine the severity of the jaundice, and whether there is likely to be an underlying problem.

How to assess

- How old is the baby, and when did the jaundice appear?
- Does the baby seem well?
- Is the baby feeding well?
- Are the nappies wet?
- What is Mum's blood group?
- Are the stools normally pigmented?

- How far down the body does the jaundice go?
- Is it getting worse, better or staying the same?

The 'must do's

☑ Always **assume that there is a serious cause if the jaundice appears in the first 24 hours.** They may be haemolysing or septic (see pitfalls).

☑ You should **treat a mildly jaundiced baby who seems uninterested in feeds, or cries excessively as a potentially ill baby.** At best, they need assessment because they won't feed well enough to get better. At worst they may have a serious infection.

☑ If jaundice is getting worse and you are unsure – refer.

☑ Always refer a baby with jaundice and abnormally pale stools – if they have biliary atresia (a condition where the biliary tree closes up over the space of weeks), time to treatment is critical.

☑ Physiological jaundice may take longer to resolve than two weeks, but by this point other causes become a concern. Refer for a 'prolonged jaundice screen'.

Pitfalls to avoid

☒ Septic babies often do not have the courtesy to look ill or have fevers. They are often just 'a bit off', feeding poorly or manifest with other such vague symptoms.

☒ Babies often don't look dehydrated, and it can be difficult to assess how well breastfed babies are feeding. Wet nappies are good, but dry nappies for longer than six hours are worrying. If in doubt, weigh the baby. The birth weight divided by their current

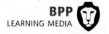

weight gives you the percentage that the baby has lost since birth, eg 2.85kg / 2.54kg = 1.12 – indicating a 12% weight loss.

☒ **Most** of that loss is fluid, so a figure of >10% represents a significantly dehydrated child even if they look well.

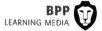

How to be a know-it-all

- Remember to consider the mother's blood group as a risk factor for haemolytic disease of the newborn. If she is blood group O or Rhesus negative then you should be more concerned. You can further ensure that you identify the babies who are at risk of haemolysis by looking at Mum's pregnancy booking blood test results, which should state whether antibodies were detected.
- Consider whether the baby was normal prior to becoming jaundiced. Are they dysmorphic? Down syndrome, for example is associated with liver disease, and syndromes can be hard to detect immediately after birth. Remember to take nothing for granted and look with fresh eyes. This will help you to pick things up that others may have missed.
- Look at growth parameters. If the baby in front of you is on the small side, and particularly if they have a small head, the cause may have been an in-utero infection (eg cytomegalovirus or 'CMV'). Considering this may prompt early referral and investigation.

A guide to the initial management of neonatal jaundice

Having said all that, most of the babies that you see will simply have mild physiological jaundice and not require treatment. If the baby looks like this:

- Well
- Alert
- Taking feeds well
- Onset of jaundice >24hrs old
- Jaundice persisting less than two weeks so far
- Wet nappies
- <10% weight loss since birth
- Pigmented stools

...then you can almost relax. All you have to do now is decide how severe the jaundice is. Even in a well baby, if a bilirubin level is above the treatment line on a phototherapy chart (see example) then your patient should have phototherapy to prevent levels reaching dangerous numbers that would potentially lead to seizures, profound deafness, cerebral palsy and even death. However it is still possible to make a clinical assessment in some cases without testing bilirubin levels.

So the first thing to do is to look at your patient without the benefit of lab tests. Do they look very yellow? If so then they should be tested to see just how high their bilirubin level is. Is the jaundice barely noticeable? In that case there may be no need to test. There are essentially two schools of thought on this.

Some clinicians feel that since clinical assessment can be wrong, all jaundiced babies should have their bilirubin levels formally checked. The NICE guidelines published in 2010 recommend that all jaundiced babies should have their bilirubin levels checked. This can be done by a transcutaneous biliometer, however, where these are unavailable then this approach would require a blood test in all cases.

Traditionally it has been common medical practice to assess babies and decide for each clinical scenario whether to do any tests. I believe that until transcutaneous biliometers are available to all clinicians assessing newborns, clinical assessment has a lot to recommend itself. There is a significant amount of anxiety and inconvenience to parents that is associated with serum testing on all jaundiced babies (which accounts for 60% of all newborns), not to mention the discomfort caused to the child. Where clinical assessment is used, it is also common practice to take two factors into account. Firstly the ethnicity of the child will affect the assessment. The more pigmented the skin, the less noticeable jaundice will be, so a lower threshold needs to be used when deciding to test these children. Secondly, the distribution of the jaundice is useful. Jaundice first appears on the face, then the chest, abdomen and finally legs. The less the spread of the jaundice the lower the bilirubin level is likely to be. As long as a baby is assessed carefully, I believe that it is still possible to decide which babies to test and which to observe and reassess daily.

De-mystifying the role of the paediatrician: what the paediatrician might do

Jaundice in the first two weeks:

- Assess and examine the baby, take a history.
- Check bilirubin (conjugated and unconjugated)
- Full blood count (FBC) and film, and reticulocyte count*
- Coombe's test for antibodies

The bilirubin level will be plotted on or checked against a bilirubin chart (see Figure 1). This will guide the decisions that need to be made regarding treatment and retesting. Note that acceptable levels are lower in the first couple of days only because hyperbilirubinemia at this stage requires action sooner to prevent any complications.

---

*Reticulocytes are the immature blood cells present in the blood stream when the bone marrow is working harder than usual. As such, if it is raised, a reticulocyte count can indicate the presence of haemolysis.

Jaundice longer than two weeks:

All of the points for the first two weeks plus...

- Check that the Guthrie test was normal
- (hypothyroidism will cause prolonged jaundice)
- Recheck thyroid function
- Full liver function tests
- Urine for culture and reducing substances
- Gal-1-put for galactosemia
- Possibly a clotting screen and many more tests besides!

FAQs

Should I suggest that a breastfeeding mother change to bottle feeding if jaundice is persisting?

The short answer to this is 'no' because you should be considering more important factors. The main concern with feeding in jaundiced babies should be 'are they getting enough?' rather than what type of milk they are having. If a baby is well hydrated and well in themselves, then there is no indication to change method of feeding. Although jaundice is more common in breastfed babies, it should be considered to be more normal in these babies as well. I would not try to list the many benefits of breastfeeding. However, should you wish to have them recounted to you, all you need do is to stop a mother from breastfeeding. The local breastfeeding police will then be obliged to remind you of the benefits of breastfeeding until you see the error of your ways. Some guidelines that I have reviewed do recommend considering the interruption of breastfeeding for 24–48 hours, but this has a significant chance of leading to a complete cessation of breastfeeding and so I would advise against this practice. If you do need to intervene, it is important that you should use the treatments which really work, rather than suspending breastfeeding. Certainly, don't interrupt breastfeeding if a baby is mildly jaundiced and well hydrated.

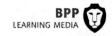

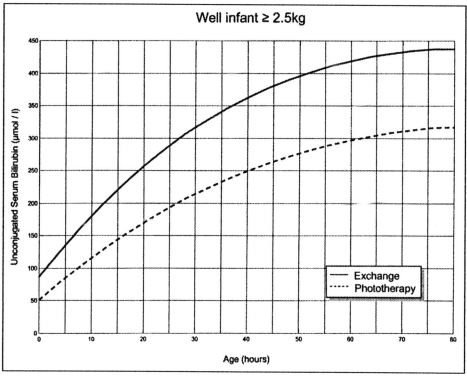

Figure 1.1 Bilirubin chart
(copyright of Dr Alan Gibson at Jessop Neonatal Unit, Sheffield Teaching Hospital
and used with his kind permission)

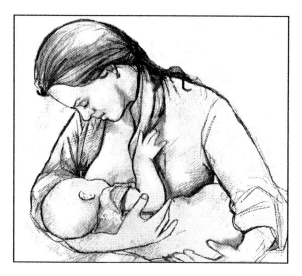

Figure 1.2 Breastfeeding mother (copyright of the
National Institute of Diabetes and Digestive and
Kidney Diseases, National Institutes of Health, and
used with their kind permission)

Also worth knowing

- Babies with pigmented skin are slightly less likely to have visible jaundice. Jaundice in these babies should further raise the index of suspicion that there may be a pathological cause.
- The bilirubin levels at which to intervene are essentially based on consensus rather than on clear evidence. In fact, this is also true of the interval for retesting. In the absence of evidence, doctors have a rare opportunity to apply common sense to make their decision of when to recheck bilirubin levels!
- Phototherapy does not always immediately lower bilirubin levels. The light alters the bilirubin to make it water soluble. This has two beneficial

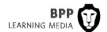

effects – it stops the converted bilirubin from passing through the blood-brain barrier and at the same time, it allows bilirubin to be cleared by the kidneys as well as by the liver. Clever, eh?

- Bilirubin binds to albumin, which is why some units use albumin boluses for severe jaundice.

What do I tell the parents?

In all cases:

"Jaundice is a word that doctors use to describe yellow skin. It is so common that almost all babies get it to some degree. Jaundice is usually not harmful. The main reason for this to appear is that newborn babies have livers that don't work very well to begin with. However, the liver will start to do its job within the first couple of weeks in most babies."

If I don't think that treatment or testing are needed:

"I don't think that the degree of jaundice your child has is a problem at the moment. Also, I am reassured by how well they are feeding and having wet nappies. We don't need to do any tests at the moment, but it is important to keep a close watch on the situation. Your baby needs to be reviewed by [you]/[GP]/[midwife] if there is more yellow colour in the skin; if your baby isn't alert and feeding well; if they seem frequently unsettled; or if their nappies aren't as wet." [You can of course make a planned review yourself or arrange to have a review made by someone else. If you expect someone else to do a review, you should speak to them first.]

If you do think that testing is needed:

"Your baby is well at the moment. I am concerned about the jaundice that they have and think that we need to test to see how high the levels are in the blood stream. This is very important because if they are high and we do not treat, then it can be harmful to your baby. If the levels are high enough to need treatment, then there are good and effective treatments for jaundice."

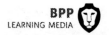

Flowchart for managing neonatal jaundice

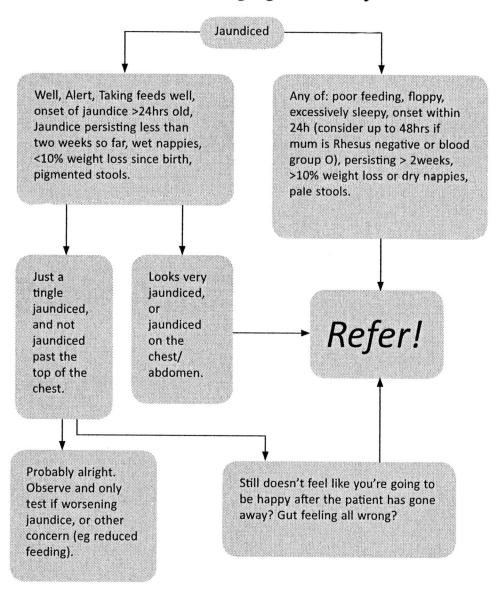

Figure 1.3 Flowchart for managing neonatal jaundice

Summary for neonatal jaundice

- Neonatal jaundice is common and usually physiological.
- Neonatal jaundice usually requires no intervention, and settles on its own.
- However, neonatal jaundice can cause neurological damage, and in severe cases, death.
- Jaundice can be caused by a variety of underlying problems, including haemolytic disease and sepsis. These cases must be managed aggressively.
- Babies with possible sepsis or haemolysis cannot simply be observed. They will deteriorate rapidly.
- Jaundice in the first 24 hours of life should always be considered pathological.
- Physiological jaundice can quickly become severe if a baby is not feeding well.
- If in doubt, arrange for bilirubin levels to be tested or refer for assessment.

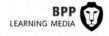

Chapter 2

Feeding and growth problems in the first year

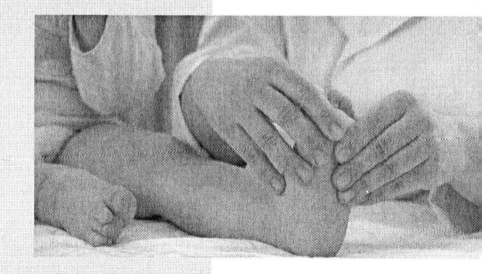

Feeding and growth problems in the first year

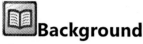

Background

This is a very common problem for GPs, and in my experience causes much confusion. Although these problems present in a primary way less often to the emergency department (ED), a thorough ED doctor will pick up on these often unnoticed problems amongst the minor illnesses and injuries. However every encounter is an opportunity to identify such problems and it is easy enough to plot a child on a growth chart. Most babies have a 'red book' or other document which contains a visual record of their growth. This can be a useful tool for identifying children who may have feeding and growth issues, but monitoring can also cause huge amounts of anxiety in parents, doctors and health visitors who all start to get palpitations when a baby crosses a line on their growth chart. The problem of trying to make a sensible assessment of the child is made worse by parents' reports of the child's feeding. I have frequently been presented with children who *never* feed, *always* vomit back the *whole* feed and more, haven't had a wet nappy for days, and have visually lost huge amounts of weight. These babies are usually smiling at me in a knowing way, while drooling and bursting out of their baby grows. You see, parents are programmed genetically to worry. So, a posit becomes 'the whole feed', and all vomiting (you will notice) is projectile. Then there may be friends and relatives who accompany the parents and choose to show support by adding to the increasing anxiety. These well-meaning people feel that it is their duty to make you see how badly this baby is wasting away. Of course, they may be correct, but in that case, it should be relatively straightforward to identify that there really is a problem.

Your task therefore is to identify the well, thriving baby in order to reassure parents and avoid inappropriate investigations. You also need to periodically identify a child who is genuinely failing to thrive. You must then determine what the underlying problem is and decide whether to refer to a paediatrician or initially intervene yourself.

How to assess

The first thing to understand is that **there is no good or universally agreed definition for faltering growth.** The way that I was taught at medical school defined the crossing down of two centiles on the growth chart as 'failure to thrive'. However this is a poor measure on its own. It is possible to lose the same amount of weight and yet cross different numbers of centile lines depending on where you started. It is therefore better to look at the growth chart as a whole for some idea of whether you should be concerned, but remember that it is only one part of the jigsaw. Remember to look **at the baby and not just the growth chart.**

The basics of assessing possible faltering growth:

- Take a history. Who is worried – the parents or health professionals? Are they feeding but not growing, or growing but not feeding?
- Ask about frequency of wet nappies.
- Ask about any watery or bloody stools.
- Ask about any family history of similar problems.
- Take a feeding history. Be specific and don't accept vague or sweeping answers.
- Plot weight, length and head circumference. Look at trends since birth.
- Examine the baby fully, as at a newborn exam.
- If a child has been small from birth and is simply tracking the centiles, check parents' heights. Are they both short?

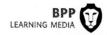

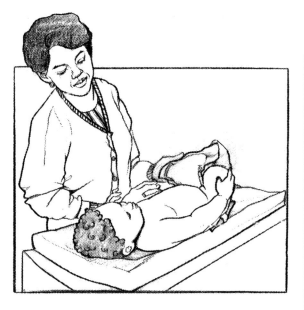

Figure 2.1 Doctor weighing baby (image provided by the National Institute of Diabetes and Digestive and Kidney Diseases, National Institutes of Health)

The 'must do's

- ☑ Look at the baby. By this I mean the baby as a whole. Do they look well? Taking a growth chart at face value without seeing the child is a fast track to embarrassment. They may be completely well and thriving, in which case you have avoided an unnecessary referral, or they may be quite unwell, in which case you will be glad that you asked to see them and didn't just refer to a routine outpatient appointment.
- ☑ Examine the baby as though they have never been examined before.
- ☑ Consider the mother's appearance. Does she look well nourished? Does she seem depressed or excessively anxious?
- ☑ Consider that there may be a medical problem, though most cases are not related to a problem with the baby, but rather a lack of calories.
- ☑ Remember to consider neglect. Both physical neglect and emotional neglect will affect growth.

Pitfalls to avoid

- ☒ Looking at the growth chart without looking at the child.
- ☒ Not checking that weights etc. have been plotted correctly.
- ☒ Accepting statements that the baby is feeding well or feeding poorly. Always ask for volumes and frequencies, or frequencies and (if applicable) whether breasts feel emptied.
- ☒ Do consider how experienced a parent is. A parent who has four other children is much more likely to know what is normal. At the same time don't fall into the trap of dismissing a first-time parent's concerns. They have instincts that are still valid.
- ☒ Thinking that all vomiting is reflux – it is often overfeeding.
- ☒ Thinking that because someone else should have by now looked at baby's palate, listened to their heart etc. there will be no point in looking again. It is best to examine the baby from scratch.

How to be a know-it-all

More than any other specialty, paediatrics is riddled with rare syndromes. Each is somewhere on a scale from rare to vanishingly rare, and you are unlikely to encounter most of them in an entire career. Paradoxically there are so many of these syndromes that you will probably encounter one unexpectedly at some point. Despite the fact that you cannot possibly learn how to recognise each one individually, you can recognise when you are seeing a child who may have a syndrome, if you keep the possibility in your mind. Feeding and growth problems are a likely presentation of many syndromes and metabolic illnesses. These conditions are often initially unrecognised, and if you are the one who spots that something is a little different, you will be at risk of feeling rather pleased with yourself.

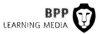

So how do you spot the rare syndrome? By noticing the unusual, which means that you need to see lots of normal children so that you will find yourself thinking 'that's odd' when something seems out of place. The important thing is to pay attention to your gut feeling, and at least discuss what you have found with a colleague.

Specifically, the kinds of thing that should make you consider one of the more unusual medical causes are listed here:

- Previous child deaths or late miscarriages in the family.
- Consanguinity of parents.
- Exposure to toxins during pregnancy (eg alcohol, recreational drugs or prescribed medication) and history of antenatal infections.
- Low birth weight and persistently low weight/length/head circumference since birth.
- Dysmorphism – this is a tricky one, and often quite subjective. Many babies do look a little odd, especially in the first few hours after birth. If a child is mildly dysmorphic then I would suggest that you look for a family resemblance first, and if there is none, then you take your findings as a whole. Allow your full assessment to take it into account, rather than giving something non-specific a lot of influence on its own. Dysmorphism on its own is a significant clue and may prompt early referral of a child with a feeding or growth problem.
- Other abnormalities such as heart murmurs should raise suspicions, because any abnormality, even if initially assumed to be benign, may suggest an underlying condition.
- The tone of the baby in particular is important. Babies with congenital abnormalities are frequently floppy.

If you think that there are indicators of an underlying syndrome then, assuming that the child is well, a paediatric outpatient follow-up should be arranged.

Finally, in the well and normal child, you should still consider the possibility of a medical problem. A urinary tract infection (UTI) is a common cause of medical failure to thrive, and may not be apparent in any other way. I believe that arranging a clean catch or pad urine specimen for those children who do not require hospital treatment is a good thing.

Also worth knowing

- Cow's milk protein intolerance (CMPI) is over-diagnosed but still an important cause of feeding and growth problems. Every effort should be made to try simple changes to feeding, before changing to specialised formulas. If a baby does seem to be convincingly affected by CMP intolerance, there are dozens of milks available to use. They work by breaking down the proteins so that they do not cause the problems that the whole protein would. The first stage is hydrolysed milks (eg 'Pepti') which have partially broken down the proteins in the milk. Some formulas go further, and contain only amino acids (eg 'neocate'). See below for further advice on management.
- Because the size of the placenta affects growth in the womb, some babies will exhibit what is referred to as 'catch down' growth in the first few weeks. They will most likely be brought to your attention by someone who is concerned that the child has dropped through two centiles. These are large babies at birth whose natural weight is on a lower centile. These babies may maintain their weight rather than gaining any, until they find the centile where they belong, which they then grow along obligingly. They are healthy throughout and do not look

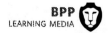

like they are failing to thrive. Another clue lies in the child's proportions. Look for symmetry of the different measurements. If weight is dropping to approximate the centile on which the length is already on, 'catch down' is more likely. If weight is dropping and falls to a centile well below that of length, then growth failure is more likely.

Convention regarding plotting measurements for premature babies is as follows:

- For babies born between 37 and 42 weeks gestation (ie 'at term'), plot their growth from the thick line that represents a term delivery ie week zero. Do not correct for gestational age when plotting measurements, instead plot as if their birth day was the same as their due date.
- For premature babies (born before 37 weeks), correct for gestational age. In other words, a baby born at 34 weeks will have their weight at 8 weeks old plotted on the line for week two in their growth chart. Continue to correct for gestational age until 24 months old.

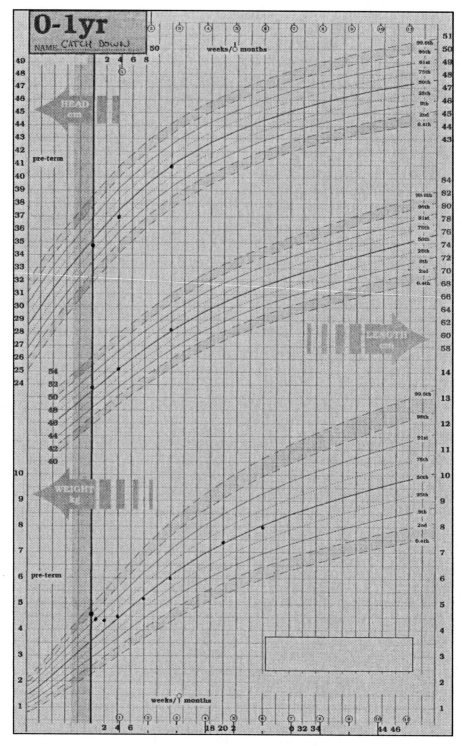

Figure 2.2a Catch down growth chart
(copyright of the Child Growth Foundation and published with their kind permission)

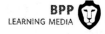

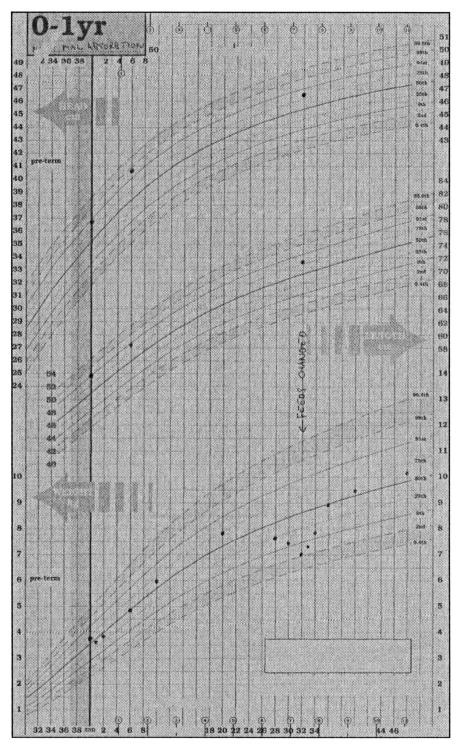

Figure 2.2b Malabsorption chart
(copyright of the Child Growth Foundation and published with their kind permission)

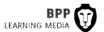

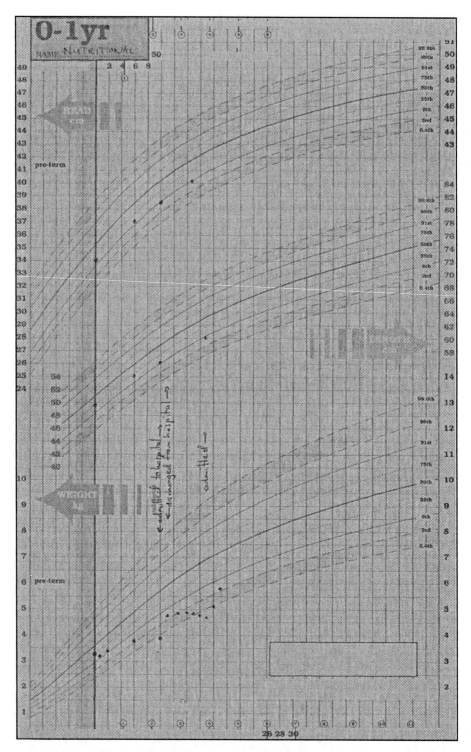

Figure 2.2c Nutritional deficiency
(copyright of the Child Growth Foundation and published with their kind permission)

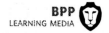

A guide to the initial management of neonatal jaundice

If the baby's weight is genuinely faltering, then a referral may be helpful. However if the child is well and you can identify a problem that may respond to intervention without the need for secondary care, you may be able to manage the problem yourself, without need for referral. (Of course, when I say 'by yourself', I mean with the backup of the full multi-disciplinary team, without whom no doctor could manage.)

Usually, by the time a GP or A&E doctor is involved, midwives and health visitors have already been involved and have attempted to address any feeding difficulties. It is definitely worth asking what interventions have been tried, and making sure that the health visitor or feeding specialist midwife has been involved (many maternity units have someone with this role, whom parents can access directly through the postnatal ward or community midwives). This is especially true for breastfeeding problems. If you are encouraging mothers to abandon breastfeeding without making efforts to help a breastfeeding mother to succeed, you will fall foul of the breastfeeding police.

Some problems can be quite straightforward to manage. If the baby is well but failing to thrive, then it may help to avoid unnecessary investigations if a specific problem can be identified. Apart from feeding difficulties, there are several underlying problems which can be initially addressed in primary care, and if successful will avoid referral altogether (Fig. 2.3).

If you feel that a baby is not as well as they should be; the weight loss is dramatic; or you have found evidence of an underlying cause that you are unable to treat, then you need to refer the child to the paediatric outpatient clinic or to the on-call team depending on the state of the child.

Problem	Clinical picture	Possible interventions
Not feeding well (a 'poor feeder')	The baby is being offered appropriate feeds but not taking adequate amounts. Not gaining adequate weight but length and head circumference are usually still increasing. Otherwise healthy on examination.	Babies who feed poorly are usually successfully managed in the community with advice from the feeding nurse/health visitor. This should include direct observation of feeding practice. Some babies need encouragement and a routine to ensure regular feeds rather than 'demand feeding'. Try orthodontic teats for bottle-fed babies. Occasionally, surgical division of tongue tie is needed (if this is present).
Not being offered enough feeds	Not gaining adequate weight, but length and head circumference are usually still growing. Otherwise healthy on examination. Only temporarily settled by a feed. These babies often spend a lot of time crying because they are hungry. When offered a feed they take it hungrily.	Advice from feeding nurse/health visitor including observation of feeding practice. Ensure understanding of the need for regular adequate feeds. Address mother's mental health, and find out what practical and financial support she has. If child protection concerns, involve a social worker and a paediatrician.

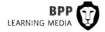

Problem	Clinical picture	Possible interventions
Reflux	Non-bilious vomiting of varying degrees. This ranges from positing, to large vomits. Vomiting may not be present is 'occult' refluxing. Crying and back arching are associated with feeds and immediately afterwards. May not be able to finish feeds due to discomfort. Faltering growth is rare and indicates more severe reflux.	Reflux tends to improve on its own given time, so non-intervention is one option if the child is thriving and feeding well. If feeding or growth is affected, treatment should be started. Ensure that there is no overfeeding. (See FAQs.) Raise head end of cot slightly. (do not advocate sleeping in car seats as there is evidence that this is harmful). Try adding thickeners/antacids to feeds if needed. Refer if severe or not responding.
Cow's milk protein (CMP) intolerance	Initially thriving and weight falling after a few weeks or months of life. Usually a family history of atopy, possibly including milk intolerance. It is common for these babies to have eczema to some degree. Note that CMP intolerance can affect breastfed babies.	This can be diagnosed and treated initially on clinical grounds, without the need for tests. If the history is suspicious with regard to CMP intolerance then changing feeds (or mother's diet for breastfed babies) on this basis alone is justified. **Do not** use soya milk, as this is likely to also cause malabsorption in these babies. Either refer, or use a hydrolysed formula for four weeks and re-challenge with ordinary formula after this. For breastfeeding mothers, a total dairy exclusion diet is mandatory. If necessary refer to a dietician, as such strict diets are hard to achieve without expert advice.
Lactose intolerance	Usually a well baby until an episode of diarrhoea +/- vomiting (gastroenteritis). The baby becomes well as the illness subsides but the diarrhoea persists and may be frothy and even pink.	Prescribe lactose-free milk for two weeks and then re-challenge with ordinary formula.
Infantile colic	**Colic is not a cause of failure to thrive**, though babies with faltering growth may also have colic. The child with isolated colic is well and thriving. They cry a lot and classically draw up their knees while doing so.	There are no longer any licensed effective treatments for infantile colic. Fortunately babies grow out of this condition, making advice and reassurance the most important part of management. (see 'what I tell parents' in chapter 6)
Significant pathology eg low grade bacterial infection, pyloric stenosis	In some cases the weight loss is just a bit more than you would expect, or the child does not seem quite right. Sometimes the vomiting is progressively worse or the feeding deteriorating.	These babies should be considered to have serious pathology and should be assessed acutely by the paediatric team. Babies especially can present in quite vague ways with significant illnesses. If in doubt, discuss with an experienced paediatrician.

Figure 2.3 Significant factors to consider for diagnosis

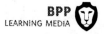

Paediatricians will be happy to get referrals like these, especially if you have been through as much of the above assessment as is practically possible.

Bloody stools are indicative of inflammation of the bowel mucosa. This suggests more significant pathology and should be referred appropriately. If there is blood in the stools then surgical causes of abdominal problems should also be considered (see Chapter 6).

 De-mystifying the role of the paediatrician: what the paediatrician might do

- Take a full history and examine the baby again.
- May admit the baby to assess feeding and to see if a couple of days of monitored feeding in hospital results in a dramatic weight gain.
- Obtain urine for culture.
- Investigate for organic causes of faltering growth unless the cause is reasonably clear. These investigations are usually in the form of multiple blood tests, urine tests, and sometimes a sweat test for cystic fibrosis.
- Probably involve various colleagues to help in the assessment, including dieticians and speech therapists who will be able to advise on nutrition and mechanics respectively.
- If reflux is failing to respond to simple antacids, an H2-blocker or a proton pump inhibitor will be started alongside a drug to improve motility (usually domperidone).
- They will not be as equipped as the GP to assess the mother's wellbeing or get a good understanding of the home circumstances. A GP can help the paediatrician enormously by writing a letter which includes this information, and phoning the doctor at the receiving end of the referral to explain any issues which are difficult to put in writing.

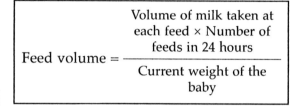 **FAQs**

How can I work out how much feed a baby is taking?

This requires a thorough history, not accepting vague answers designed to reassure. With formula-fed babies, the feed volumes can be calculated if you know: how large the bottles are that the baby is offered, how much the baby actually takes, the number of feeds in a 24 hour period and the current weight of the baby.

$$\text{Feed volume} = \frac{\text{Volume of milk taken at each feed} \times \text{Number of feeds in 24 hours}}{\text{Current weight of the baby}}$$

Volume taken is in ml (1 fluid ounce = 28 ml)
Weight is in kg
Feed volume is then in ml/kg/day

Of course, when a baby is partly, or exclusively breastfed, this calculation doesn't help you. However you can still get an idea of whether a baby is feeding adequately. The important thing to avoid doing is asking 'does your baby feed well?' and being happy with the answer 'yes'. Breastfeeding is not always easy, and I feel that we often unfairly expect mothers to know whether it is 'going well'. If they have landed in a consultation with you, there is a significant likelihood that feeding is not adequate, so I recommend the following questions to give you a more objective assessment (all answers should be 'yes'):

- Do your breasts ache before feeding, and is that relieved by a feed?
- Do your breasts leak milk before a feed, or when your baby cries?
- Does your baby have properly wet nappies several times a day?

If a breastfeeding baby is vomiting after a feed then the feed is likely to be adequate. The

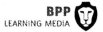

vomiting itself then needs to be assessed and consideration given as to whether the baby has reflux or another problem.

What is a normal feed volume for a baby?

The somewhat obtuse answer to this is simply that each baby is different, and that many normal babies take 'abnormal' feed volumes but thrive despite this. However, assuming that we are applying this question to a baby who is either not feeding well or not growing properly, we need to apply some judgement regarding whether this particular child's feeds need adjusting.

The average newborn gets very little fluid in the first few days (thus the initial weight loss) but should be taking about 60ml/kg/day on day one, rising to around 150ml/kg/day by day five. Feed volumes stay at this level for the first few months and then gradually tail off until the child grows into a feed volume of 100 ml/kg/day by about six months old. Of course, the total volume increases throughout due to the phenomenal growth that babies achieve in the first year.

There is no chart available with standard deviations and normal values of feeds at different ages, so in the absence of a tool, you will need to apply judgement. I believe that the first test of whether a feed is the correct volume is dependent on whether there is a problem. If there is no problem, leave well alone.

If a feed seems too great or too small, then that needs to be put in context with the problem. If I find that a baby who is failing to thrive and vomits but takes 200mls/kg of formula, then I would probably advise reducing feed volumes to 150ml/kg/day. And if a one-month-old, who was otherwise well, was failing to gain adequate weight on 150ml/kg/day, then I might suggest increasing to 165ml/kg/day. One would not normally advise increasing feeds beyond 180mls/kg/day.

So, the real answer is, there is no 'normal' volume of feeds – but you can usually deduce if a baby may be underfed or overfed, based on a simple calculation and the overall picture, and then advise accordingly.

What do I tell the parents?

When someone is concerned that a baby is not gaining weight, or not taking enough feeds, yet the baby is thriving and well:

"All babies are different and feed differently. Having had a good look at your baby's growth charts, and examined your baby, I am very reassured. Your baby is growing well and seems to be a normal healthy baby. I understand that you were concerned, however since your baby is growing as they should be, they must be getting the nutrition that they need to grow. You should continue to do what you are already doing from the point of view of feeding. If something changes and you have new concerns, we may need to see your baby again but otherwise it is fine for them to continue and be weighed as and when the health visitor recommends."

When a formula-fed baby (prior to weaning) is not gaining adequate weight and I feel that increasing feeds would help:

"Your baby's growth charts show that they are not gaining weight as well as we would expect. Having examined your baby, they seem otherwise healthy. This makes it most likely that they need a few extra calories to give them the additional energy that will help them to grow. The best way to do this is to try increasing their feeds. [This can be done either by increasing volume or frequency and will depend on what you have calculated as the target feed volume.] A small increase in calories will usually make a significant difference to growth. We will check your baby's weight again in one week to be sure that this change has helped. If not we will need to consider whether your baby needs any tests or treatments."

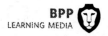

Flowchart for assessing feeding and growth problems in the first year

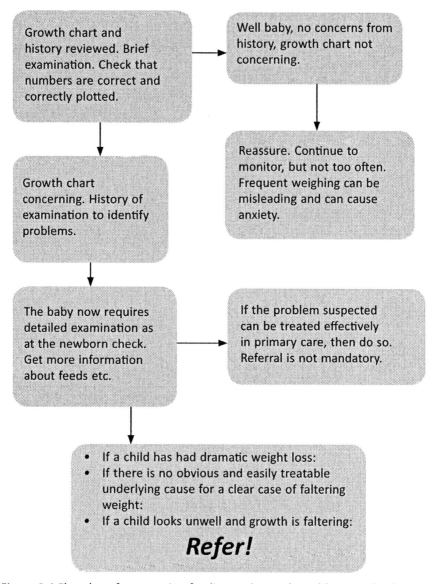

Figure 2.4 Flowchart for assessing feeding and growth problems in the first year

Summary for feeding and growth problems

- Faltering growth can be easily misdiagnosed by plotting measurements wrongly.
- Poor weight gain and feeding problems in a child who is well can often be initially assessed and treated in primary care.
- Poor weight gain in a child with any concerning signs or symptoms should be referred to a paediatrician.
- A thorough examination is essential to properly assess children with faltering growth.
- A thorough feeding history is essential to assess babies who present with growth or feeding problems.
- Many babies who have been considered to have a feeding problem have growth charts that clearly show that they do not.
- If a baby is thriving then they must be taking and absorbing adequate feeds.

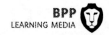

Chapter 3

The coughing, wheezing or snuffly child

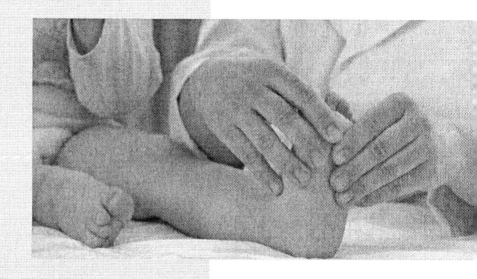

The coughing, wheezing or snuffly child

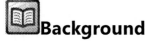## Background

If you haven't already seen uncountable numbers of preschool children with coughs and wheezing and everything that can go with a viral illness, then the bad news is that you will. Catching viral coughs and colds is a normal part of growing up. There is even evidence that doing so helps the immune system to develop healthily and may reduce a child's chances of becoming atopic. For the parent, however, it can seem to be a disaster when their child catches a cold. You are usually faced with a barrage of hyperbole by whoever accompanies the child:

- 'He can't breathe, doctor' or
- 'She won't eat/drink/walk' etc.

You shouldn't be put off at this point by the fact that the child may be smiling at you (while they empty your sharps bin onto your desk, which they have nimbly climbed onto). This is not Munchausen's by proxy that you are faced with but a parent who needs your help and reassurance.

Many children in these circumstances are prescribed antibiotics, or inhalers, or steroids, when often no such treatment is needed nor would be helpful. Now, I know *you* would never do this but some doctors feel pressured in these circumstances to give something so the parents feel that they have been taken seriously. Sadly, this approach doesn't work. Prescribing unnecessary treatments causes parents to re-attend more often and takes the emphasis away from the simple over-the-counter medication that is genuinely effective for these children. If you're having a really unlucky day, they might even have a bad reaction to the treatment (that you administered in the hope that you might be preventing an 'early pneumonia'). Worse still, if you are the doctor who tends to prescribe more,

these snotty children will prefer to come to see you more often and tend to avoid your colleagues who prefer explanation and reassurance to antibiotics as a rule. Do not fall into this trap; instead aim to treat those who will benefit from treatment and avoid unnecessary medication where possible.

In order to know which child to treat and what to treat them with, you will need to make a working diagnosis. This process is more of an art than a science. Knowing which are the important signs and symptoms to give weight to is the most important part of getting it right. There is no way to be right all the time with this group of children, but you can greatly improve your accuracy by learning to focus on certain factors and give less weight to other signs and symptoms.

How to assess

- **Do they look well? Are they breathing comfortably?** This initial 'eyeballing' of the child will give you the best assessment of whether they should worry you or not. From there on, you are working towards a specific diagnosis, while remaining open-minded that your initial assessment may need to change in the light of further information.
- Have they had a fever? If so was it severe (>39°C)?
- Have they had any floppy or blue episodes?
- Have they had any treatments (eg medicine, inhalers)? Did they help?
- Have they had previous episodes of this problem?
- Do they have any symptoms between episodes (eg cough, wheeze, nocturnal or exercise-related symptoms)?

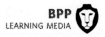

- Do any of the parents or carers smoke? If so, when are they stopping?
- Is there a family history of asthma/ eczema/hayfever?
- Examine the ears and throat.
- Examine the chest and cardiovascular system.
- Are they well hydrated?
- Are they playing/cheerful, or subdued?

It is important to note that assessing respiratory problems requires the clinician to sometimes act on information as they gather it. The first point of assessment is the 'Do they look well?' question. If the answer is no, then it is inappropriate to get as far as asking about pets before examining the child. In the cases where you find yourself faced with a significantly distressed child, ask about symptoms, onset, and medication (including allergies) before examining the child to assess the cause of the distress and the efficacy of breathing. Wheezing is almost unique in medicine because, no matter where you are, you can administer emergency therapy and once this rescue medication is started, a detailed history can be taken.

Any child who is given a treatment for their breathing or circulation should be reassessed within ten minutes from such an intervention. Here is a golden opportunity to do so at no inconvenience. If you are seeing a wheezy child over twelve months old, give inhalers or nebulisers if they are obviously needed and then take a full history. Then, when you have finished, you will be ready to do a more thorough examination. By doing a before and after examination you can determine whether your initial treatment has helped.

I would also encourage brevity in reaching the point of deciding that a child needs referral. It is clumsy to rush to the phone before having enough important information to be able to make a good referral; however, I do not believe that the child's interests are served by taking an overly detailed history, despite an obvious need to get help from the paediatric team. I am aware, of course, that all GPs and emergency medicine doctors can recall a story about referring a child who is going blue, only to have a paediatrician ask for details about which particular breed of parrot the child has as a pet. Please be polite in these circumstances. The doctor at the other end of the phone has been reading too many books, and knowledge of minutia is a hazard of being a hospital medic. In the meantime, you are, of course, doing your job well if you haven't established that the child has a Brazilian long-tailed parrot before making the referral.

The 'must do's

For the sake of emphasis, I am going to give just one 'must do' for this section, albeit a big one. When a child presents with a respiratory problem, parents will tend to put a great deal of emphasis on the cough and the wheeze. Although these are useful clues as to what you are dealing with, they are common symptoms in quite well children. You should be considering not the presence of such symptoms but the effect which they are having. In other words, the **cough, wheeze or ruttle are not nearly as important as the child's degree of respiratory distress or general unwellness.**

Remember:

- ☑ Respiratory distress should be considered an early warning sign that, eventually, the child may deteriorate and potentially do so rapidly.
- ☑ When a child shows signs of reduced efficacy of breathing, this is a sign of impending disaster.

(See the section at the beginning for a guide to assessing work and adequacy of breathing.)

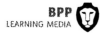

Pitfalls to avoid

- ☒ Do not allow yourself to forget your initial impression. If the child looks well, then they probably are. If they look unwell, then try to assess how badly and consider why the child has become unwell. Of course it is also appropriate to act on the additional information you gather. For example a six-month-old may look well, however even if they clinically have just a cold, if the parent tells you that the child had an episode where they went blue at home, (ie had an apparent life-threatening episode) they should be observed and further assessed by an experienced paediatrician.

- ☒ Accepting someone's initial description of symptoms at face value can be very misleading. What do they mean by a 'wheeze'? Experience tells us that people mean many different things when they refer to a 'wheeze'. Make sure that the parent or child understands the question, and that you understand the answer. Can they do an impression or description of what the 'wheeze' sounds like for you?

- ☒ Always keep an open mind after your initial assessment when it comes to chests. Due to the frequency with which circumstances change and new symptoms develop, it is good to 'keep the door open' for children with respiratory symptoms. It is imperative to make a confident clinical decision to begin with but also to be aware that, for example, bacterial pneumonias are often preceded by a viral upper respiratory tract infection. I find that the safest solution to this potential for change is to tell the parents what they should expect to happen.

Then they can come back if something changes and the child's clinical course takes an unexpected turn.

- ☒ **Bronchiolitis is not routinely complicated by secondary bacterial infection.** The vast majority of the babies with bronchiolitis (even the ones who are poorly enough to need hospital treatment) do not benefit from antibiotics. Giving these children antibiotics 'just in case' makes their feeding worse and may further dehydrate them by giving them diarrhoea.

- ☒ **Mistaking focal signs for pneumonia is a very common mistake in children.** Children with any respiratory infection often have crackles focally in their chest. This is due to intermittent mucous plugging, rather than true pneumonia in most cases. If a child has pneumonia, you will be able to tell that this is the case by the fact that they have a significant fever, a cough, respiratory distress and are unwell to some degree. If they are snotty but well and have no respiratory distress then you can usually ignore focal crackles.

- ☒ Thinking that a clear chest rules out pneumonia is just as likely to lead to a wrong diagnosis. In fact, **the unwell looking child with fever, cough and respiratory distress should make you very suspicious of pneumonia, even if you cannot hear any focal chest signs**.

- ☒ Not looking properly at the ears and throat will leave you without a vital piece of the jigsaw. An ear, nose and throat (ENT) examination is definitely a challenge in some children, but by not doing a good ENT examination, you will be missing important signs.

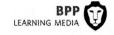

You should now have all the information that you need to make an assessment and decide how to manage the child. Wait a second though. It's still very easy to put too much emphasis on the wrong findings. Much of the process of assessing these children is counter-intuitive and although it is tempting for example to treat crackles heard in a chest, you should become comfortable with the idea that these can be very misleading. Bizarrely enough, your assessment of the chest from the outside is probably more consistent than your assessment with the stethoscope. So I have produced some generic patients who will, I am sure, be familiar to you. With them is my suggested approach for how to manage each patient group.

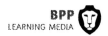

Flowchart for classifying wheezy children

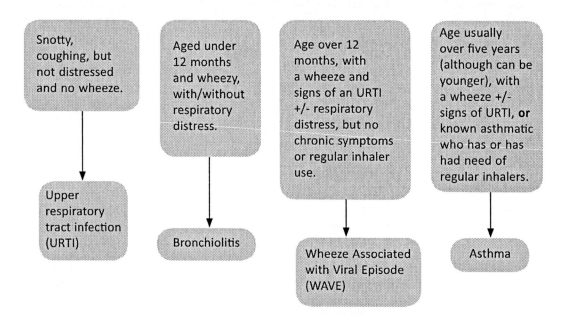

'The how to be right almost all the time' guide to classifying wheezy children

Use this flowchart to choose which treatment pathway is most appropriate for your patient. Bear in mind that there is considerable overlap and blurring between these categorisations. They are useful to decide on a starting point but a good clinician always keeps an open mind about the diagnosis.

Snotty, coughing, but not distressed and no wheeze.

Aged under 12 months and wheezy, with/without respiratory distress.

Age over 12 months, with a wheeze and signs of an URTI +/- respiratory distress, but no chronic symptoms or regular inhaler use.

Age usually over five years (although can be younger), with a wheeze +/- signs of URTI, **or** known asthmatic who has or has had need of regular inhalers.

Upper respiratory tract infection (URTI)

Bronchiolitis

Wheeze Associated with Viral Episode (WAVE)

Asthma

For any of the above groups, a fever above 39°C is highly suspicious of a bacterial infection, although viral infections can also produce high temperatures. The triad of cough, fever and respiratory distress should be considered a lower respiratory tract infection until proven otherwise (see Chapter 5). Also look for other foci of infection – ears, throat, urine or other. **Remember that sepsis of any origin can cause tachypnoea, tachycardia and grunting and so mimic respiratory distress.**

Finally, consider foreign body inhalation at all ages, and hyperventilation (usually in the context of an anxiety attack) in the older child.

Figure 3.1 Flowchart for classifying wheezy children

Once you have decided which group your child best fits into, use that as a starting point for further assessment and management. It is preferable not to diagnose asthma too readily since many asthma treatments are not effective for other causes of wheeze. However, consider this: these conditions all represent different manifestations of similar processes. This is especially true of wheeze associated viral episodes (WAVE) and asthma. Being absolutely certain of which of these is the correct diagnosis is not always necessary. Treating the respiratory distress is the first priority, which will be in the form of bronchodilators for WAVE and asthma and with oxygen (if available) for bronchiolitis, as well as severe WAVE or asthma. In the acute setting, the exact diagnosis matters less than treating symptoms. The classification may well be best kept as 'wheezy/viral episode' until a pattern emerges, at which point the specific diagnosis will help to guide long term treatment.

The following sections provide approaches to treating the various subgroups outlined in figure 5. If a bacterial lower respiratory tract infection is suspected, this is covered in Chapter 5.

3.1 The upper respiratory tract infection (URTI)

Assessment

This is what to expect when a child has an upper respiratory tract infection (URTI):

- Any age.
- Looks well, though may be miserable.
- No respiratory distress (though children may breathe quickly when febrile and be significantly tachycardic, this resolves with the fever unless there is also true distress.)

- Fever usually <39°C and responds well to paracetamol +/- ibuprofen.
- Snotty, inflamed ears or pharynx/tonsils.
- May have a non-specific blanching rash.
- May have crackles in the chest. These are likely to be transmitted from the upper airways. They are often intermittent. Only if they sound like true crepitations, and are consistent and focal, should they lead you to a diagnosis of pneumonia when a child has an apparent URTI. Also look for other signs that you would expect in a child with pneumonia: poor air entry or dullness. If respiratory distress is absent, pneumonia is unlikely.
- If the child is cheerful, active, playing and especially if they have not had a fever, you can be fairly confident that they do not have pneumonia.

Management

- Reassure. But don't say 'it's *just* a virus' unless you want a sleep-deprived parent to start crying in your consulting room.
- Explain that these infections are a normal part of childhood, and will happen frequently (about twelve per year for many children) and that these infections strengthen the immune system.
- Encourage fluids (if possible, not sugar free drinks – sick children need calories!) and paracetamol +/- ibuprofen.
- Explain that the infection may take days to clear but as long as their child is slowly improving, they should continue to let the recovery period take as long as it needs.
- Any viral URTI can be a precursor to a bacterial infection, so warn them that sometimes other infections develop. Request that if their child seems worse despite their medicines, they should get the child seen again.

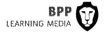

De-mystifying the role of the paediatrician: what the paediatrician might do

- Paediatricians also see children with uncomplicated URTI. The management in secondary care should be no different to that in a general practice or emergency department setting.
- In my experience there are two common reasons for children to be seen with URTI sib secondary care.
  The first is that the child has been seen by a doctor who has not found a focus for the fever. In these cases it is simply a matter of a more determined doctor looking in the ears and throat.

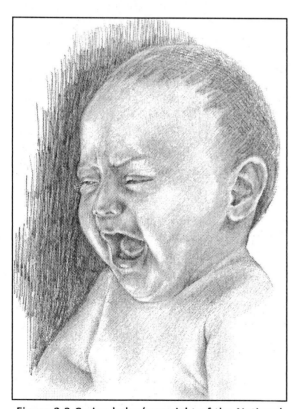

Figure 3.2 Crying baby (copyright of the National Institute of Diabetes and Digestive and Kidney Diseases, National Institutes of Health, and used with their kind permission). Acute ear pain is a common cause of inconsolable crying.

The second reason is that an unexpected rash has appeared on the child's skin. They are otherwise well and have all the signs of a URTI. Most of these rashes are non-specific but some have occasional petechiae. In the case of the latter, a period of observation is advisable, even if the end result is that the clinician – experienced enough to do – so decides that the rash is due to a viral infection.

How to be a know-it-all

- Not all earache is otitis media. Any URTI can block the Eustachian tube. This causes a difference in ear pressure that can be quite painful. The best way to determine true otitis media is to convincingly see a bulging, inflamed, dull tympanic membrane. A perforation and discharge is also a give-away. Even if there is a pink ear drum, if the tympanic membrane is shiny, then Eustachian tube blockage is more likely and so antibiotics are not indicated.
- Because they are very common infections, there are rarely circumstances where an URTI is apparent, but something else is going on. However, because URTIs are so much a fact of life for children that the chances of a child having one when they develop something unrelated are very high. In other words, **just because the child has signs of a URTI does not mean that they do not have another infection elsewhere.** So in order to be a clever doctor, you need to consider the child who presents with unusual signs and symptoms, yet has signs of an URTI, as possibly having a second pathology. Especially worth considering is a urinary tract infection (UTI). UTI is more common around the time of URTIs because the antibiotics which have been given, albeit well-meaningly, can encourage urinary tract infections to develop.

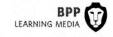

- Conversely, consider the child who does present with unrelated symptoms, and yet no-one can find a cause. For example, a three–year-old complains of tummy pain yet no pathology has been found, because, so far, doctors have been examining only what seemed to them to be the relevant part of the child. Because children are peculiar beings, ear pain can manifest as a miserable child, an abdominal pain or headache. There is nothing quite so satisfying (except perhaps lancing a boil) as being the first doctor to bother to look in this child's ears or throat. When you find a tense, red, bulging tympanic membrane or massive tonsillitis, you can explain that children often complain of abdominal pain, or head pain, or any pain for that matter, when in fact the pain is coming from their ears or throat.

Also worth knowing

- For the first few months of life, babies are obligate nose-breathers. This is thought to be an arrangement designed to prevent choking. If the mouth is involved with anything, the baby is programmed to swallow. If breathing is required, this must come from the nostrils. This effect is so strongly programmed that a newborn who has congenitally blocked nasal passages (choanal atresia) will be completely unable to breathe without help. Similarly, but thankfully not so dangerously, if you are unlucky enough to be a few weeks old and catch a cold, you will struggle. Babies can look quite distressed with nothing more than a snuffly nose to cause their troubles. With a baby who is more than just a few weeks old, has no risk factors (eg prematurity, heart disease) and is otherwise well, it can be worth getting a friendly nurse to do some gentle nasal suction (if the facilities are available). If this completely resolves the distress then you are able to reassure and advise. If the baby is very small, then 'snotty and distressed' is still unlikely to be harmful, but you may wish to refer the very little babies for observation on the grounds that they may have early bronchiolitis.

- While we often worry about minor infections progressing to more severe infections, we sometimes forget that minor illnesses can be serious for other reasons. One example is that children occasionally develop hypoglycaemia during a URTI or episodes of diarrhoea and vomiting. Children consume large amounts of energy during viral illnesses, especially when they have a fever. When their liver glycogen is all consumed, they rapidly become hypoglycaemic. This is why **a child who is suffering with any infection and suddenly becomes drowsy should always have a blood sugar checked.** Also be aware that in order to correct this, only oral, buccal or intravenous (IV) sugar will work since glycogen stores have been exhausted.

- It is sometimes reasonable to refer a baby for paediatric assessment, even if you are happy with the baby. One possible reason for this is unfavourable social circumstances. That doesn't have to mean that you are concerned at a child protection level, though this could of course be the case. Anyone can find themselves with their child looked after in hospital for 'social reasons'. If for example you saw a professional couple who were first-time parents, with a snotty two-week–old, and they had just moved house, the boiler had broken and the phones weren't connected, with no local support network… well, you could just reassure them and send them on their way but you probably should offer referral for

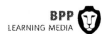

further assessment. (As emphasised elsewhere in this book, please do not tell the parents that you are *admitting* them. Circumstances may change and your paediatric colleagues will make the final decision as to whether further observation is indicated.)

FAQs

When should I give antibiotics?

There are a quite a few things in medicine which are rather subjective, allowing the doctor to make the findings fit the outcome that they have already decided on. Ears, chests and throats are three of the most common examples. If you really want to give antibiotics to a child, it is fairly easy to find an excuse to do so.

However, there is a wealth of evidence that most childhood infections are viral and that even when respiratory tract infections are bacterial, they usually resolve without treatment and respond disappointingly to antibiotics. At the same time, we know that a proportion of these children go on to develop serious and even life-threatening illnesses. There is no doubt that antibiotics should be used in a subgroup of children with upper and lower respiratory tract infections. The number of potential complications of streptococcal infections is endless, and yet most children with streptococcal infections do not develop any complications. So how do we decide when to give antibiotics to a child for what is likely to resolve without treatment?

Firstly, I believe that **swabs should essentially** *never* **be used to decide whether to treat in the context of minor illnesses**. I also feel that they are rarely needed to guide treatment, though they do have a role here, particularly in screening for certain infections when you really need to know what you are treating, such as when treating conjunctivitis in a newborn baby. Essentially, I believe that **you should decide clinically whether to give antibiotics**. If you test, and wait for the result of the swab to determine

the need for treatment, the result is likely to be unhelpful and too late to be relevant. What will you do when you get a result several days later showing that something has grown from your swab? By now the child is probably better and if the child has not improved you should have advised them to get reviewed when they failed to do so after a few days.

Instead I use a simple two stage approach to deciding whether to use antibiotics for a sore throat and/or ear infection:

1. Firstly, does the child appear toxic? I realise that this is a subjective term and may not even be a legitimate medical word in this context. However, some children are not septic but just have that 'more-than-just-a-bit-unwell' look to them. I give these children antibiotics.
2. Secondly, I ask myself whether the illness is responding to simple medicines such as paracetamol and ibuprofen in age- and weight-appropriate doses, given at regular intervals. If not, I believe it is time to reach for the broad spectrum antibiotic (which you have just checked that the child is not allergic to, yes?).

I realise that there is no science to back this approach but it does come with grade 2b evidence: 'I've always done this and to my knowledge it has never gone wrong.'

This child seems to be having too many minor illnesses. How many infections can a normal child have?

Many books will give a flat answer that 12 to 15 minor illnesses every year is an acceptable rate of infections in early childhood. To make a sensible assessment however requires a little time considering the whole child. True immunodeficiency is uncommon in childhood.

Most children who are having frequent infections are doing what normal children do. They develop immunity by becoming infected. This is an important part of maturing the immune system and the end result is beneficial. If not exposed to infections in childhood then the consequences include greater likelihood of becoming atopic. In some cases it is actually safer to have certain infections as a child. For example, if you catch chickenpox (varicella) for the first time in adulthood, your immune system is no longer in its heightened, developing state so the infection affects you much more severely than having it as a child.

To get an idea as to whether a child is having an abnormal number of minor infections then I would consider the following:

- Is the child thriving and developing normally? If not then underlying immunodeficiency is more likely.
- Consider the frequency of infections but be aware that you cannot really expect anyone to be accurate when you ask questions of this sort. Instead you might need to accept that parents will give us a number because you have asked for one, and that it can be used to get an idea of how many infections it feels like the child has had.
- Has the child had even a couple of significant infections (bacterial infections requiring hospital admission)? Especially if these have progressed to complications, then multiple infections such as pneumonia and cellulitis should raise your suspicion that the child may have an immunodeficiency.
- Is there a good explanation for a period of repeated infections? Probably the most common example is the child who has started nursery a few months previously. These children then get infection after infection after infection before suggesting to the GP that there may be something wrong with the child's immune system. However, the clue is there in the timing of the illnesses, and the fact that the child was well prior to starting nursery. Thankfully, acquired immunodeficiency in children is very rare in the UK, so children who are

initially well and then later start to have repeated infections rarely have an underlying immunodeficiency.

What do I tell the parents?

When I have diagnosed a URTI:

"Having examined your child, I am pleased to say that I have not found any signs of serious infections. Your child has all the signs of a cold/sore throat/ear infection, but their chest is clear. Because the tubes to the chest are shorter in children, any mucous in the nose or throat can make it seem like there is a problem in the chest. The kind of infection will usually last a few days and because most of them are viral, antibiotics are just as likely to cause problems (such as diarrhoea) as they are to help. The main aim with treating this kind of infection is to make your child feel as well as possible until they fight the infection off. I can't tell you how long that will take exactly, but children will only be this unwell with a cold/sore throat/ear infection for a couple of days usually. After that the child will usually get better in themselves over the space of a few days, though they may be snuffly and have a cough for a lot longer."

"It is important to make sure that they drink plenty of fluids, and while they are ill I would advise avoiding sugar-free drinks. Water is fine if that is what they will drink, but a weak sugary drink of some kind, such as diluted fruit cordial, is even better. Do not worry if your child doesn't feel like eating, as long as they are drinking well. Regular paracetamol and/or ibuprofen will help to control any temperature and make them feel more like their usual selves. As long as you don't exceed the amount recommended on the bottle, you can keep giving these until your child seems better. If you are unsure about what medicines to give, it is always best to ask for advice."

"These infections happen a lot in childhood and sometimes children go from one infection to another. However if your child seems very unwell despite doing all the things we have talked about then you should bring them to be seen again. In particular, if they are working hard to breathe, or seem floppy or drowsy, you should make sure you get them assessed

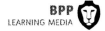

as soon as possible. If your child seems significantly worse, it is likely that there is a new problem on top of this illness."

"I am quite happy that your child is well enough to go home at the moment but you should not hesitate to bring them to be checked again ,if something becomes worse or doesn't get better when it should have done."

Flowchart for assessing the child with an upper respiratory tract infection (URTI)

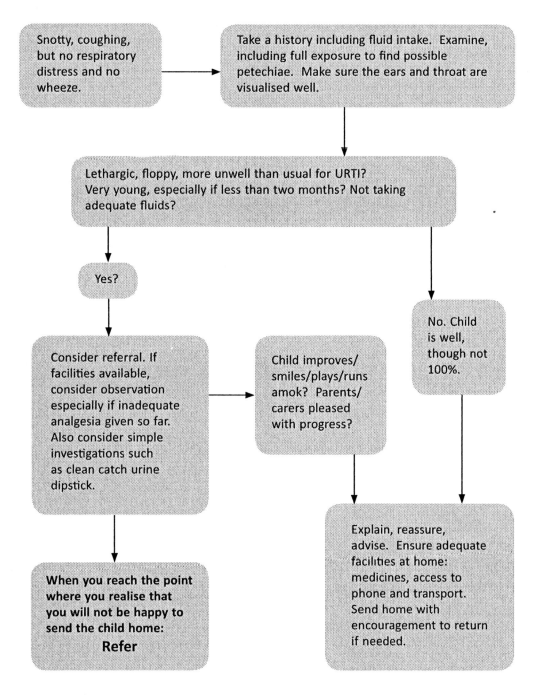

Figure 3.3 Flowchart for assessing the child with an upper respiratory tract infection (URTI)

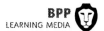

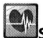

Summary for upper respiratory tract infection (URTI)

- In a child with cough, coryza, sore throat, or painful ears then URTI is most likely.
- It is easy to allow chest auscultation to mislead you. In the absence of respiratory distress and a significant fever, lower respiratory tract infection is unlikely.
- Adequate analgesia will suffice in most cases and may also demonstrate how well the child can be during a period of observation and further assessment.
- With patients who are seen and sent home, remember that you are only seeing a snapshot of how they are. Listen to the parents and make sure that they feel that they could bring their child back for further assessment.
- A child with an apparent URTI may later develop a more serious infection. The early stages of some serious illnesses may have the same signs and symptoms as an URTI. Always keep the door open for reassessment.

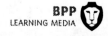

3.2 The bronchiolitic baby

Assessment

Basic criteria for likely bronchiolitis:

- Age from a few weeks to around twelve months old.
- Tight, wet, high-pitched cough.
- Wheeze.
- Fine crepitations.

Further information:

- Does the child look well?
- Is there respiratory distress? Is it mild, moderate or severe?
- Is the baby febrile? (If temp >38°C then simple bronchiolitis is less likely.)
- Is the baby drinking well?
- Is the baby well hydrated? (Wet nappies and wet mucous membranes.)
- Does the baby have other lung problems (eg prematurity)?
- Is there good air entry throughout on auscultation?
- Has the baby had any apnoeas or blue episodes?
- Are the parents able to cope and seek further attention if needed?

Management

- Hospital admission for bronchiolitis is usually to support feeding or because the baby needs oxygen therapy for respiratory distress. **If the baby is well hydrated, only mildly distressed, and there are no other worrying findings in the history or examination, then it is reasonable to allow the baby home.** Advise the parents that no medication helps, and that they should allow the baby to take smaller feeds more often. If anything worsens they should seek a medical review.
- If there is significant distress (eg respiratory rate >60 breaths per minute, moderate recession, looks tired), poor feeding, dehydration or anything complicating an otherwise straightforward bronchiolitis, then I would advise referral.
- **I would advise against giving babies with bronchiolitis steroids or antibiotics.** Steroids do not help and are to be avoided when possible under the age of 12 months old. Bacterial infection does not commonly complicate bronchiolitis infections. As for a URTI, it is easy to misinterpret the chest signs of these babies as being indicative of pneumonia. If a baby does have bacterial infection on top of bronchiolitis then they could get very unwell indeed, so I feel that sending a child home on antibiotics is inadvisable, as well as generally unnecessary for bronchiolitis. **If you feel the baby you are seeing is well enough to go home they are very unlikely to have a bacterial pneumonia.**
- Ipratropium inhalers don't always help but do little harm either.

De-mystifying the role of the paediatrician: what the paediatrician might do

- Each child is assessed on their own merits as above. Many children are allowed home with advice about when to seek reassessment. In most cases blood tests and X-rays do not add useful further information.
- Essentially there are only three ways that secondary care can manage bronchiolitis actively.
  1. Some children will be feeding poorly enough to need their oral feeds supported. This is done by frequent small nasogastric bolus feeds. If the child is recessing severely then intravenous fluids may be preferred.
  2. If the child has low oxygen saturations then supplementary oxygen is given, often by nasal cannula.

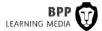

3. In the most severe cases, the child will reach a point where due to severity or exhaustion, respiratory failure necessitates ventilatory support and high dependency unit/ intensive care unit admission.

How to be a know-it-all

- Firstly, learn to recognise the cough. There are only a few conditions that can be diagnosed with reasonable reliability by recognising a particular sign. The distinctive cough of bronchiolitis is one example, and the sound of it quickly becomes familiar when heard a few times. It sounds moist, it has a 'tight' sound to it as you would expect with airways constriction, and it is high-pitched. Another way to describe it is as though a sneeze came out as a cough. When you recognise this cough, you can start to recognise bronchiolitis before the wheeze or crepitations have appeared, which can be very useful indeed.

- Know that bronchiolitis tends to follow a reasonably predictable pattern. Usually it starts with a cough and coryza and then gets worse over the space of three or four days. However bad it is then, the child usually goes through a plateau phase for three to four days, getting no worse and no better. Then the worst symptoms resolve over a few days, often leaving a well child with a nuisance cough and a tendency to wheeze whenever they catch a cold. This pattern is useful to know for three reasons.
  1. You can advise parents about what to expect.
  2. It will help you to make sensible clinical decisions. For example, if a baby is borderline for referral on day two, you are more likely to refer than if they are borderline on day

seven of the illness, when they are about to get better.
  3. It helps you to spot the unexpected. If a child with bronchiolitis is getting worse on day seven, you should wonder why. Could they be developing a secondary bacterial infection?

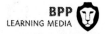

Also worth knowing

As is always the case, there is a rarer condition which can catch out the unwary, yet presents with almost identical signs and symptoms. **Heart failure** (due to, for example, a large ventricular septal defect or 'VSD') **presents in the same age group as bronchiolitis.** It can even be the case that the fact that a baby was born with a heart problem, which has been undetected until they develop a simple coryzal illness. This extra cardiovascular strain then precipitates acute heart failure. Thus the baby presents with a coryza coupled with the respiratory distress and poor feeding that is normally classic bronchiolitis.

Frustratingly, babies with heart failure don't have the courtesy to demonstrate specific clues at first assessment. The typical baby with cardiac failure may present with quite vague symptoms such as poor feeding. On examination they may have a wheeze and possibly fine crepitations in the chest. Again, this is not very helpful in distinguishing heart failure from bronchiolitis since both conditions share all these signs and symptoms.

So how do you recognise these babies from among the rafts of bronchiolitic babies who come every winter? The answer follows a common theme in paediatrics: your gut feeling about the child will be that something is not quite right, and when you know what to look for you might find some evidence to confirm your anxieties. If in doubt, ask a colleague to review the baby. The main clue should be a mismatch between any cardiovascular compromise and the respiratory compromise. Bronchiolitic babies can become so unwell that they are poorly perfused, but this is usually preceded by at least moderate and usually quite marked respiratory distress. Conversely, 'cardiac' babies will develop respiratory distress but this is secondary to the cardiac failure. So the babies to be suspicious of are the ones with mild respiratory distress but quite high pulse rates and prolonged capillary refills. They may have a heart murmur, weak or absent femoral pulses and they may have sacral oedema. There may also be major clues in the history. It may be that their 'hole in the heart' is well known to the parents and they may be waiting to see the heart specialist.

So, while you should not start imagining that every baby with respiratory distress, wheezing and poor feeding has heart failure instead of bronchiolitis, you should be aware that one day, you may see one that does.

 FAQs

Why do different inhalers work sometimes but not others?

If we are to stand any chance of giving effective treatment, it is a good idea to understand how the different inhalers work. Then by matching the inhaler to the disease process, you are more likely to see the benefits and to understand the reasons for not seeing any improvement.

Salbutamol and other short-acting β-agonists work by relaxing smooth muscle in the bronchial tree. It is therefore an excellent drug to treat bronchospasm. Bronchospasm is the process which is present in asthma exacerbations, to a lesser extent during viral wheezing and probably not at all during bronchiolitis. The airway constriction in bronchiolitis consists mainly of oedema and secretions rather than bronchospasm. Note that smooth muscle tone in the bronchial tree is actually important to babies, who have a tendency to have floppy airways until they develop strong cartilage rings. It is possible therefore to make conditions

such as bronchomalacia (see Chapter 4) worse with β-agonists. This is because, rather than constricting the airways, the smooth muscle helps to support the airway. β-agonists relax the smooth muscles which in theory could make matters worse.

Agents such as ipratropium work primarily by drying secretions. This is probably why they have traditionally been used for bronchiolitis (where the wheeze is due to exudate in the lumen of the bronchioles rather than bronchospasm). However, the evidence for benefits is conflicting. These drugs also help the degree to which secretions worsen viral wheezing and asthma. However, to treat true bronchospasm adequately, β-agonists are the drug of choice.

It is good practice to reassess any child after giving inhaled bronchodilators to appraise the benefit. Of course, in clinical practice, the whole issue of whether an inhaler was effective is usually subjective. Even if the clinician is diligent enough to reassess the child after a dose of inhalers it can be difficult know whether they have helped. The placebo effect of giving an inhaler (which affects the parents, doctors and nurses more than the child sometimes) is substantial, which only adds to this difficulty.

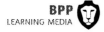 **What do I tell the parents?**

When a baby has bronchiolitis but does not need admission to hospital:

"Your baby has all the signs of a condition called bronchiolitis. This condition is a lot like when you have a cough with a cold. The difference is that because the tubes are so small in babies' chests, the small amount of swelling caused by the virus makes it difficult for them to breathe. The difficulty breathing can also cause them to struggle with feeding. At the moment, your baby is managing to cope well enough so that I do not feel that they need support with breathing or feeding in hospital."

"There is no treatment that works well for the infection itself. Usually it follows a fairly predicable

pattern of getting worse over 3–4 days, then staying the same for 3–4 days and then getting better. The cough often stays for many days, but your baby should be otherwise well. It is also possible that when your baby gets further colds, they may get the same problem again."

"If your baby has more trouble breathing or doesn't feed well then we may need to help them with that. I am happy for you to take your baby home. You should offer them small feeds frequently and allow them to refuse a feed if they are tired. If their breathing gets worse, they are having poor feeds or dry nappies, you should get them seen again. The best person to tell if anything is wrong is you, so do not worry that people might think that you are an anxious parent. If you feel that something is wrong, you will be correct most of the time so do not ignore your concerns."

When a baby has bronchiolitis, and needs admission to hospital:

"Your baby has all the signs of a condition called bronchiolitis. This is a lot like when you have a cough with a cold. Because the tubes are so small in babies' chests, the small amount of swelling caused by the virus makes it difficult for them to breathe. The difficulty in breathing can also cause them to struggle with feeding."

"I think that your baby is really getting tired with the difficulty they are having with their breathing. Because of this, we should get them seen by a paediatrician. They can then decide whether to help breathing with some oxygen. Sometimes the paediatricians also need to help with feeding by putting a tube through the nose into the stomach so that they can give them milk that way. This rests your baby, allowing them to breathe more easily and still get their milk."

Flowchart for assessing babies with bronchiolitis

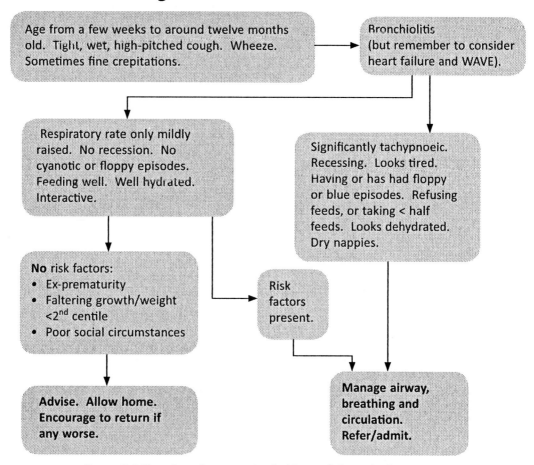

Figure 3.4 Flowchart for assessing babies with bronchiolitis

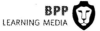
Summary for the bronchiolitic baby

- Bronchiolitis is a common condition which occurs almost exclusively during the first year of life.
- Cases occur in epidemics during the winter months but also sporadically during the rest of the year.
- Babies with bronchiolitis usually start with a typical cough and develop wheezing, poor feeding and respiratory distress.
- Most babies do not need to be assessed or treated by a paediatrician.
- The mainstay of hospital treatment is supportive (nasal oxygen, nasogastric tube feeding)
- Babies who are well enough to be managed at home are unlikely to have bacterial lower respiratory tract infection and should not be prescribed antibiotics.
- Babies whose breathing or feeding is significantly affected require assessment with a view to supportive treatment.

3.3 The wheeze associated with viral infection episodes (WAVE)

Assessment

Basic criteria for WAVE:

- Age usually around twelve months to five years but may be slightly younger or older.
- As well as being coryzal, has a tight cough.
- Wheezing.

Further information:

- Is there respiratory distress? If so is it mild, moderate, severe?
- Is the child well?
- Is the child looking tired?
- Is the child febrile? (if temperature >38.5°C then a simple viral infection is less likely)
- Have they had wheezy episodes before?
- What worked last time?
- Have they already tried anything for this episode?
- Is there good air entry throughout? Remember that as a wheeze gets worse it gets quieter and ultimately becomes a silent chest. So listen carefully to decide whether there is good air movement in the chest.
- Consider other diagnoses: specifically, an inhaled foreign body and anaphylaxis. To screen for these ask about choking episodes (which may be days ago) and look for swelling around the lips and urticaria.
- Check oxygen saturations if available but always look at the result as extra information, rather than starting with the saturations as the basis for the assessment.

Management

- If the diagnosis appears to be a wheeze brought on by a viral illness, there is no more than mild distress and the child has not had to take large doses of bronchodilators at home, then you can try the child with 6–10 puffs of salbutamol through a spacer. If they respond well, it is likely to be safe to allow the child home to have four puffs of salbutamol hourly until the episode passes.
- If you have had a good response to inhalers, you may want to observe to see how long the effect of the inhalers lasts. This is particularly important if the child is younger, having their first episode or worst episode of wheeze. In a GP setting, 'observing' may simply mean bringing them back in a couple of hours to be seen again. In hospital, it means keeping them in your department for a couple of hours.
- Oral steroids for mild cases are somewhat controversial. Experience suggests that they work but there is evidence that they don't. I still use steroids for viral wheezers but less than I used to.
- If the child is really distressed, properly unwell, tired or has already had lots of inhalers (effectively) then even if they respond to initial treatment, I would advise referral.
- Although the name suggests a benign condition, these 'viral wheezers' can have life threatening episodes. Essentially, the acute management for these children is the same as for an exacerbation of asthma. You need to assess the severity of the episode and treat accordingly (see British Thoracic Society guidelines in any British National Formulary). Giving adequate inhaled therapy as soon as possible makes the most difference.
- If a child is unwell enough to require a doctor to give them a stat dose of inhalers or a nebuliser, then I believe that the same child should be reviewed by that same doctor five to ten minutes after the inhaler to see what effect the treatment has had. This will help you and the child enormously. If you do this then you will gain vital information and in most cases, be able to document an improvement. Not uncommonly however, you will find no improvement, or even

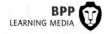

deterioration. In these situations, you are potentially dealing with a seriously ill child and it is important to repeat the dose of salbutamol, while monitoring the child carefully and considering escalating the level of care.

- In a GP setting, requiring a second dose in quick succession should prompt rapid referral to secondary care. Careful consideration should be given as to whether the child should go by ambulance. If the child looks significantly distressed or unwell then they may require referral even if they respond to treatment.
- **As a rule, it is better to give more bronchodilator than less**, as long as you recognise that the more you give, the more seriously you should take the child's illness. In other words, if you give a 5mg salbutamol nebuliser to a four-year-old with a wheeze, then you should not then turn around and send them home when their wheeze settles.
- In the emergency department, you should follow departmental guidelines as to how much treatment it is reasonable to give before referring. If in doubt, discuss with a colleague in the department or on the paediatric team.
- Don't forget that this is an opportunity to suggest that the parents stop smoking. URTIs and wheezy episodes are both more common in children where there is a smoker living in the house. Note that the presence of smokers in the house is the risk factor (not just smokers smoking in the house) and this needs explaining to parents who say 'I smoke, but never in the house.' (See 'what do I tell the parents?' below.)

De-mystifying the role of the paediatrician: what the paediatrician might do

- Wheeze associated viral infection episodes are a common reason for admission to paediatric units.

- There is little place for investigation in these children and most are assessed purely clinically.
- Most cases are managed with simple inhaled bronchodilators with or without systemic steroids.
- Most paediatricians would avoid inhaled steroids for children who only wheeze during viral illnesses.

How to be a know-it-all

- Because children have smaller bronchi, it is possible for a wheeze to be absent with only moderate bronchospasm. One of the best ways to show your familiarity with wheezy children is to produce a wheezy child where no wheeze has yet been heard. **If a child over the age of one year old comes to you with respiratory distress and no fever, and yet no wheeze can be heard, then the diagnosis is still most likely to be bronchospasm.** So if after a brief history and examination, you ever find yourself or a colleague wondering why the child they have just seen is so breathless, I suggest trying a healthy dose of salbutamol. 'But they have no wheeze', you might reply. However, soon after your prescribed salbutamol, a wheeze will most likely appear miraculously. You see, the reason why there was no wheeze when the child was first examined was the lack of sufficient air flow to produce the characteristic whistle. Then, by giving a bronchodilator, you will improve air flow and the wheeze will appear. Of course, you need your history and examination to be thorough enough to exclude important conditions such as pneumothorax, anaphylaxis and pneumonia. So use this trial of inhalers, and if it works, people will be impressed, while if no improvement ensues, you can consider this a valuable piece of information nevertheless.

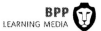

- Because children are prone to do stupid things and then not tell anyone (or of course simply not yet be able to talk), they rarely present with a history of inhaling a foreign body. Therefore, it always seems to impress when you ask knowingly 'has your child choked on anything recently?' and a parent suddenly recalls that, yes, just before the wheezing started someone in the household lost a one carat diamond ring. 'How did you know that, doctor?' they will probably ask. Well, mainly you asked because you always ask this when a child presents with a cough. You are after all a very thorough doctor, and children, as mentioned above, have a tendency to put thing in their mouths and then inhale them. The important thing is to ask the question as though you think you are on to something, especially if you have begun to suspect that this is not really a viral associated wheeze. If you have found a unilateral wheeze on examination after bronchodilators, then even if no one thinks that the child has swallowed, inhaled or choked on anything (and the child is not coryzal), get a chest X-ray.

Also worth knowing

- Sometimes children go blue around the lips during a fever. If you can establish that only the lips changed colour, either during or just prior to a fever, then this is probably not a true cyanotic spell.
- Wheeze itself is not the enemy. A child with a mild wheeze and severe respiratory distress should be considered a medical emergency. By the same token, it is possible to have a child with a severe wheeze who runs around playing cheerfully. It is reasonable to allow a child to continue to wheeze if improvement in the child's respiratory

distress is satisfactory. Treating until the wheeze is completely gone is preferable, but not always possible. In these circumstances it may be safe to permit a wheeze and treat distress only, as long as the child is visibly active and well.

FAQs

What is the difference between viral wheezing and bronchiolitis? When should I use salbutamol and when should I use ipratropium?

This question highlights that everything to do with wheezy and viral children is on a spectrum. Babies with bronchiolitis are, when they are older, re-classified as wheeze associated viral episodes and later still may be presenting with the same cough and wheeze but diagnosed as a viral exacerbation of asthma. **What you *call* an episode does not affect whether the patient will respond to treatment.** However correctly placing your patient into one of these groups does at least help to predict with some accuracy whether a child will benefit from a particular intervention. This is because the disease processes vary slightly, and so different treatments are more likely to be successful or unhelpful depending on why the child is wheezing.

Bronchiolitis is the viral wheezing, if you like, of the under-one-year-olds. Their bronchi and bronchioles are small and exquisitely sensitive to any swelling. At the same time, the 'march of atopy' (eczema→asthma→hayfever) is not usually yet in its respiratory phase so there is **unlikely to be a response to β-agonists.** Clever doctors tell me that under the age of one, babies have only just begun to develop the β receptors that will allow drugs like salbutamol to have much effect. This has led to the use of drugs such as ipratropium in bronchiolitis. Ipratropium may have some small effect by reducing secretions, but depending on the study that you look at, the benefit varies from little to none and some feel that ipratropium can be harmful. I do not personally believe that the benefits justify its routine use in bronchiolitis. However, if it seems worth attempting, a trial of ipratropium is one possible tactic. Again, I feel this needs to be trialled in each child and the effect assessed. I do not think that there is much value in giving a prescription for inhalers to the parents, unless the method is demonstrated and the benefits are evaluated.

The term for wheeze associated with viral infection episodes (WAVE) is preferred for pre-school children who present with a wheeze and an upper respiratory tract infection (URTI). This group are usually past the age where bronchiolitis best describes the presenting syndrome, but there is some overlap. For example, an eleven-month-old who presents with a wheeze and coryza might have either. In these cases it is a question of making a clinical judgement, which should include considering the question, 'does it matter which I diagnose?' If in doubt, stop agonising over the diagnosis and try some inhaled therapy.

With wheeze associated with a viral infection episode, inhaled therapy not only should work, but is also the most important part of treatment. **β agonists work quickly and more dramatically than inhalers such as ipratropium.** If they do not work, the next step is usually to give more, ensuring adequate delivery, rather than changing drug. Most guidelines include giving ipratropium as an additional drug when β agonists are not working well enough. For the reasons listed above however, the very young 'viral wheezer' may actually respond better to ipratropium. Ultimately, the process of giving one or the other and then reassessing will help the clinician to decide upon the best treatment for that child.

Finally, by the time a child is old enough to have demonstrated a clear tendency to wheeze, they may either be diagnosed as asthmatics or viral episodic wheezers. In an episode of acute wheeze, the decision as to whether to give oral steroids will depend on a previous diagnosis of asthma, or on the child having other atopic conditions, a family history and interval symptoms not related to viral episodes. Again, the particular label given is helpful mainly in deciding on a threshold for giving treatment. Rightly or wrongly, I think that the severity of the episode will influence the decision to use oral steroids. For this reason, children with severe episodes of viral-induced wheeze are rarely managed without oral steroids. However, it is more likely that true asthmatics will respond to systemic steroids in an exacerbation than a child who only wheezes with viral illnesses.

Do inhaled steroids work for viral-induced wheezes?

There is plentiful conflicting evidence to confuse the clinician in making this decision. As a result, practices vary and I suspect that doctors tend to follow example more than evidence. However, it is an important question to answer because if steroids work then we want to use them, and if steroids don't work, we don't want to give them to children.

Children who experience a wheeze only in the context of upper respiratory tract infections do not, as a rule, benefit from inhaled steroids as prophylaxis (preventative medicine). To be included in this group of viral episodic wheezers it is important to have no interval symptoms: chronic cough, nocturnal symptoms, exercise induced wheeze or seasonal rhinitis.

The difficulty can arise when a child gets cold after cold and so never recovers in between enough to be clear whether they do have symptom-free intervals. To these children I would give a five-day course of systemic steroids and then maintain them on a medium dose (for their age) steroid inhaler for 3–6 months. I would review them half way through and at the end of that period assess what the child was like on the brown inhaler and a couple of weeks after it was stopped. I would also be clear with the parents why I was doing this. Remember that if you prescribe inhalers to anyone, they or

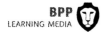

their parents will assume that they have asthma unless you explain otherwise.

With regard to systemic steroids for a virally induced wheeze, I try to reserve these for the more severe episodes. I think that it is reasonable to say that the evidence supports a strategy of using moderate amounts of β-agonist four times an hour, and, if more than this is needed, adding steroids, increasing inhaled therapy and referring where appropriate.

What do I tell the parents?

When I have decided that the child probably has a WAVE and they are not severely unwell:

"Your child has a wheeze in their chest, which means a whistling noise, which is there because the tubes in their lungs have become tight. This often happens when children get colds because the virus makes the lining of the tubes get swollen. Although this doesn't mean that your child has asthma, the treatment that helps the wheeze is the same as we use in asthma, so we will start by giving your child an inhaler through a plastic bubble to try to settle the breathing down. It is important that we make sure that your child can breathe easily before we decide that it is safe for them to go home. So I need to see how well they respond to the inhalers and then we can decide if your child needs any more treatment. Usually, I aim to get the child to the point where they only need inhalers ever four hours or so before I consider them well enough to go home."

When they have told me that they are smokers:

"Colds and wheezy episodes are much more common in children who have a smoker who lives in the house. I agree that smoking outside has got to be better than smoking inside the house. However, even when you smoke outside, your clothes are smoky and you breathe out the chemicals from the smoke for a long time afterwards."

"I realise that stopping smoking is very difficult but it is very worthwhile. People who manage to stop smoking feel much better and you and your children will be much healthier, not to mention that the money you save will make you richer!"

"If you do want to stop smoking then getting help from your GP, health visitor or pharmacist will increase your chances of success by four times or more. Don't give up trying, even if you have tried before and started smoking again. It takes an average of seven attempts before most people finally stop forever because it is very difficult. The most important first step is deciding to stop."

When I am sending home a child who has had a WAVE:

"I am pleased with the way that your child has responded to medication. Now that their breathing has settled down, if you are happy with how they are, we can talk about letting you take them home. If you are happy with how to give the inhalers, and know the things to look out for then it should be safe to take your child home. It is unlikely that they will deteriorate but it is important that you are able to get back here if your child gets worse. These are the things to look out for: breathing becoming faster, wheezing that doesn't go away when you give the inhalers, wheezing which comes back quickly after giving the inhalers and if your child looks like they are finding it difficult to breathe. You will usually know when your child is getting worse. You should trust your instincts because they are usually right. If you are unsure, it is best to seek advice by phoning us or coming back. No one will mind if you do so, and you don't need to worry about anybody thinking that you are an anxious parent."

"In particular, if your child seems to be tired, by which I mean physically exhausted because of struggling to breathe, rather than 'sleepy tired', then you should call for an ambulance. It is also a good idea if they are struggling with their breathing to give them ten puffs of their inhaler through their spacer device as well as getting help."

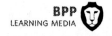

"It may take a few days for the cold to go, but the wheeze and difficulty in breathing usually only last a couple of days. If it is going on for longer, then it is a good idea to see your GP to get your child checked over again. As the breathing and wheeze settle down, you can use the inhaler less frequently and then stop. The inhaler will not help the runny nose. It is however fine to give medicines for a fever as well as the inhaler. However, if your child has a very high fever or seem really poorly, they should be seen again to make sure they aren't developing a chest infection."

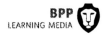

Flowchart for managing wheeze associated viral infection episodes (WAVE)

Note that this is simply a guide to how to approach a viral wheezing child. The flowchart below can be used to direct assessment and management, however it is not meant to replace local or national guidelines. I suggest that this flowchart is used to gain an overview to managing these children.

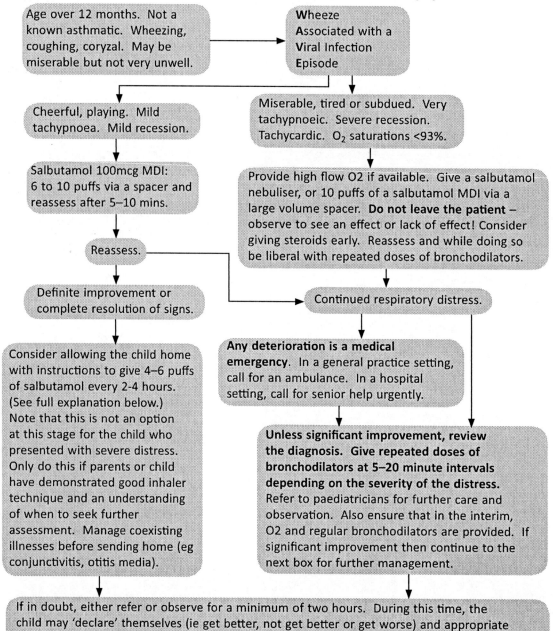

Figure 3.5 Flowchart for managing wheeze associated viral episodes (WAVE)

BPP
LEARNING MEDIA

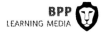

Summary for wheeze associated with viral infection episodes (WAVE)

- Children commonly wheeze during a viral URTI and this tendency on its own does not equate to being asthmatic.
- The acute disease process causing the wheeze is similar to that in asthma and so the same treatments will usually work (though probably less so for steroid medicines and inhalers)
- The children with WAVE usually have a mild respiratory distress and require only β-agonist bronchodilator treatment.
- Some children develop severe respiratory distress, require large amounts of bronchodilators and a period of observation, and are usually given systemic steroids.
- Occasionally wheeze will be absent. It is often worth trying a dose of salbutamol for children with respiratory distress who do not have wheeze and do not clinically have pneumonia.
- As a rule, it is better to give more bronchodilator than less, as long as you recognise that the more you give, the more seriously you should take the child's illness.
- The most important factors to consider are the work of breathing that the child is doing (respiratory rate, recession, using accessory muscles, air entry and ability to speak), and the efficacy of breathing (level of consciousness, tone, heart rate and energy levels). The degree of wheeze itself is also important, but secondary to these other factors.

3.4 Asthma

Assessment of acute asthma

Assessment of the acute asthma exacerbation is essentially the same as for the acute wheeze but with a few additions. The child with a diagnosis of asthma often presents with that diagnosis already known, but of course, every asthmatic has a first episode and these can be spectacularly severe. Most children though, will have had previous episodes and someone is able to tell you that they are asthmatic.

Conversely, you should also be aware that many parents believe their child to have asthma because they have been prescribed inhalers in the past. This assumption is understandable and as a result the basis for the child's diagnosis should preferably be briefly explored when possible. With a little exploration it is usually easy enough to quickly establish which children are the true asthmatics and which have had wheezy viral episodes. However, in the acute episode where time does not permit detailed inquisition, a wheeze is a wheeze and respiratory distress is respiratory distress, so the immediate management is basically the same for WAVE and asthma. To do the asthmatic justice there are just a few extra considerations, and so the management of acute asthma has been outlined below in more detail than for viral wheeze. There is also a section on the subtleties of managing the chronic aspect of asthma. To begin with, this is the information which you need to gather:

You are probably dealing with an acute asthma episode if the child has the following:

- A wheeze, or acute respiratory distress with poor air entry in the chest, and:
- They are a known asthmatic or have recurrent wheezy episodes and a significant past or family history of atopy.

- **Beware the silent chest – quiet or absent wheeze can mean severe bronchospasm if accompanied by respiratory distress.**

Then assess the following:

- If needed, start giving oxygen and inhalers before taking a full history and examining the child.
- Is there respiratory distress? If so is it mild, moderate or severe?
- Is the child well?
- Does the child look tired?
- Check oxygen saturations if available, but always look at the result as extra information, rather than starting with the saturations as the basis for the assessment.
- Ask about fever and cough.
- Consider other diagnoses: specifically an inhaled foreign body and anaphylaxis. To screen for these ask about choking episodes (which may be days ago) and look for swelling around the lips, as well as for urticaria.
- Ask about medication given at home. Does the child have a preventer inhaler? Do they use it every day? How much reliever inhaler have they been taking today, and how frequently?
- Ask about how long the child has been diagnosed with asthma. How often do they have exacerbations? How many times have they had systemic steroids in the past three months? How severe was their worst episode? How does this one compare to their worst ever episode?
- When appropriate, check inhaler technique. Never assume that a child who has had asthma for a long time can use their inhalers correctly.
- Ask about smokers in the household (see advice to smokers in the previous WAVE section)
- Ask about precipitants to this episode. Common culprits are:
  - Viral infections
  - Sudden change in the weather
  - Animals

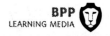

- Change in environment (eg moving house/city/country)
- Foods (however be wary of anaphylaxis – if a wheeze develops and is felt to have been precipitated by food, then a full blown allergic reaction should be suspected)

- Examine thoroughly looking for:
  - Work and efficacy of breathing
  - Any rash, especially eczema or urticaria
  - Signs of chronic uncontrolled asthma: Harrison's sulcus and pectus excavatum (see below)
  - ENT examination
  - Listen to the chest, but be wary of over-interpreting localised signs. Mucous plugging is almost always present in an asthma attack. Focal crepitations without fever or dullness should not cause you to rush to prescribe antibiotics or to request a chest X-ray.

The 'must do's

☑ Learn to rely on work of breathing and efficacy of breathing, especially adequacy of air entry and degree of hypoxia, as the factors which determine the clinical situation.

☑ Give a dose of bronchodilator that matches the child's size and severity of the episode.

☑ Always check inhaler technique at some point.

☑ Advise about the evils of smoking if needed.

Pitfalls to avoid

☒ Do not give a bronchodilator and assume that it has helped. Assess the effect shortly afterwards.

☒ Do not get caught out by a pneumothorax. Children with asthma get air trapping and so are prone to developing pneumothoraces.

☒ Do not be over reliant on chest X-rays. A trial of bronchodilator is a better assessment tool in children with respiratory distress who do not have significant fever.

Grading the severity of acute asthma

In order to determine how to manage the acute asthma attack, a decision needs to be made regarding the severity of the episode. This is not as easy in children as it is in adults. Many children cannot, for example, complete full sentences simply because they have not learned to do so yet rather than because their shortness of breath prevents them. Also, the degree to which they are frightened by being in a strange place or confident with strangers will radically affect the assessment of an individual child. When a child is crying, this can make wheeze and recessions considerably worse. Perversely however, when a child is crying this in itself is not as worrying as the child who seems too exhausted to complain, since a crying child must have more energy and reserves than a child too subdued and tired to cry. In many cases, determining the severity of a wheezy episode is not simple.

However difficult it may be, in order to proceed, a preliminary decision needs to be made. The clinician should be reassured that **most children present with mild attacks**. Also, although it is possible to have two doctors look at one child and have one decide 'mild' while the other decides 'moderate', I think that **when you see a severe episode you will recognise it as such**. Ultimately, it is best to make a decision which errs on the side of caution. If you find that the episode is a difficult one to classify go for the moderate over the mild and the severe over the moderate. As a word of reassurance, providing that the child is appropriately observed and reassessed, a misleading initial assessment would not end in disaster since moderate exacerbations do not tend to respond adequately

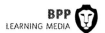

Guide to classifying the severity of an acute asthma episode

Mild	Moderate	Severe
• No significant tachypnoea • No obvious increased work of breathing • Able to speak or cry without difficulty • SaO_2 >94% • Wheezy but well • Alert and not floppy	• Mild tachypnoea (respiratory rate up to ten above normal levels) • Some increased work of breathing and use of accessory muscles • Able to talk even if slightly breathless • SaO_2 91–94% • Alert and not floppy	• Significant tachypnoea (respiratory rate up more than ten above normal levels) or slow laboured breathing • Increased work of breathing and use of accessory muscles • Unable to talk or cry comfortably • Poor air entry/silent chest • SaO_2 <91% • Subdued and/or floppy • Looks unwell and physically exhausted

Figure 3.6 Guide to classifying the severity of an acute asthma episode

to the treatment that you would give for a mild episode of acute asthma.

3.4.1 Management of mild acute asthma

A mild episode will usually be managed by the family or the child themselves. Therefore, if the child presents for medical assessment, careful consideration should be given to why they have not been successfully managed despite the mildness of the episode. The most common preventable reason for failure to respond to bronchodilators is ineffective delivery of inhalers. The reasons for this happening range from inhalers running out to poor technique and inadequate dosage. It is important to address any such inadequate delivery of bronchodilators, as failure to do so will result in a temporary improvement while in your care but an inevitable recurrence of symptoms after sending the child home. To adequately assess as to whether a child is receiving their inhalers in an effective

way, I recommend that direct questions are posed regarding the what, when, how, and the amount of treatment given in the 24 hours prior to assessment. Then, ask the carer and/or child to give the first dose of bronchodilator while you or a nurse watches, in order to assess the technique that is being used. This is often quite an enlightening experience.

It is often the case that by giving a child who is suffering from a mild asthma episode 4–6 puffs of a salbutamol 100 mcg metered dose inhaler (MDI), complete (though temporary) resolution of signs and symptoms occurs. If satisfactory improvement occurs with administration of such small quantities of bronchodilators, then it is likely that the child will do well. At this point I would advise the following:

• **Address any factor that contributed to the child presenting for assessment** (lack of confidence managing their asthma, poor technique etc).

Good inhaler (with large volume spacer) technique:

- Check that the inhaler has some medication in it by giving it a shake and feeling the medication move inside.
- Use a clean, drip dried spacer (towel drying causes static and reduces the aerosol delivery).
- Place the inhaler into its slot and the spacer into the mouth, or use a mask with a good seal on the child's face. If the child is unwilling, get extra help to both hold the child and to provide nice distractions.
- Ideally, press the button on the inhaler just before inspiration.
- Take ten deep breaths from the spacer.
- Then remove the inhaler, shake it again and repeat the process.

Figure 3.7 Guide to good inhaler technique

- **Ensure that the child has enough bronchodilator at home to see them through** (a standard MDI contains 200 doses, so will last eight days if being used at a rate of four puffs every four hours)
- **Check that the carers are clear about when to give extra inhalers and when to call for help.** Check that they have access to a phone.
- **Advise them to give the salbutamol at a dose of four puffs every four hours.** If the child fails to respond or deteriorates within two hours of the last dose, the responsible adult should give the child ten puffs of salbutamol via a spacer and get the child seen again urgently by any route possible.
- If the issue arises, **advise that steroid tablets are not required at this stage** but may be needed if the episode is not resolving within a couple of days or gets worse within that time.

- Use the opportunity to **advise the parents about modifying avoidable factors** which will make a difference to the child's asthma. The most important factor is often the avoidance of exposure to tobacco smoke.
- Treat any additional problems. Then, if there are no barriers to doing so, allow the child home. If there is concern regarding any of the above, arrange for a period of observation and reassessment of up to four hours (in the emergency department for example, or if in general practice, by arranging a reassessment of the child in surgery later on), after which time the child may well now be discharged home.

Failure of the child's signs and symptoms to respond should prompt the clinician to consider what other disease processes may be going on. Is there infection, an inhaled foreign body or an allergic reaction for example? However, if the first dose of bronchodilator fails to make a significant improvement, it is more likely that the child is still having an uncomplicated asthma episode and that the inadequacy of the initial therapy is the next piece of the jigsaw. As mentioned above, many children who present with mild episodes respond dramatically to a simple dose of 4–6 puffs of salbutamol, which may be because they were not getting this effectively so far. Those that fail to respond to initial bronchodilator therapy have now demonstrated that they may well have been having adequate treatment before they presented, and have been failing to respond to this. They may even appear to be 'mild' due to the partial response which they have had from therapy prior to seeing you. As a result, any child who fails to respond to initial treatment for a mild exacerbation of asthma should be managed as for a moderate episode.

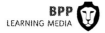

Flowchart for managing mild acute asthma

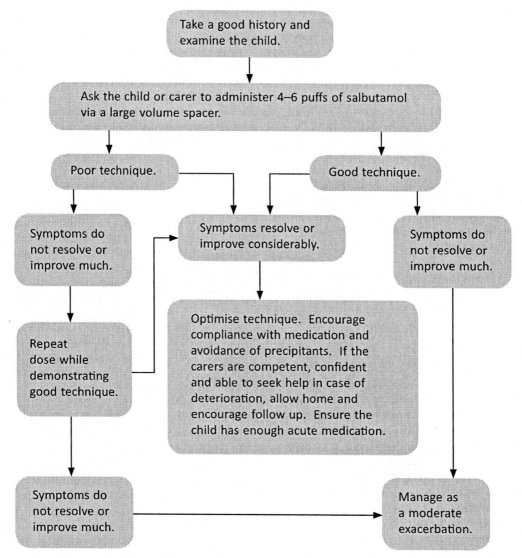

Figure 3.8 Flowchart for managing mild acute asthma

3.4.2 Management of moderate acute asthma

Moderate episodes of acute asthma should be considered as potentially developing into severe, life-threatening episodes. Once there are signs consistent with a moderately severe episode, there is the potential for a vicious cycle to develop. This occurs because the bronchospasm which is affecting the child's airways now has the potential to reduce the delivery of inhaled bronchodilators. This in turn allows the bronchospasm to worsen. The key to preventing and reversing this deterioration is the early administration of adequate doses of bronchodilators.

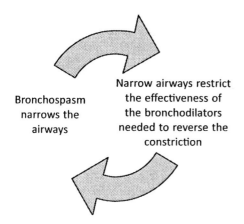

Figure 3.9 Why more inhaler is needed for worsening asthma

Since children with moderate exacerbations of asthma are not cyanosed, salbutamol can still be given via inhaler and a large volume spacer. This dose should be increased however to 10 puffs of a 100mcg MDI. This dose can then be repeated every 15–20 minutes until three doses have been given. During this time, the child should be watched carefully in case of deterioration. In the emergency department or assessment unit, this means being in clear view of a nursing station. In a general practice setting, this means having the GP sit with them while they have their treatment. During this time, urgent referral can be arranged and the child will hopefully be on their way to your

friendly paediatric unit before all three initial doses are complete.

The three initial 'rescue' doses of salbutamol advised above act to reverse the vicious cycle of poor air entry leading to reduced treatment efficacy. Each dose opens the airways a little more and by following each dose quickly by another bolus of bronchodilator, the effect is usually dramatic improvement.

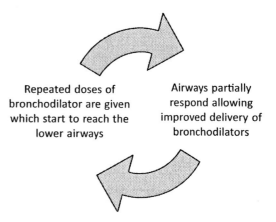

Figure 3.10 The response to good delivery of bronchodilators

Following this improvement the child can go on to continued regular treatment, usually in the form of 6–10 puffs of salbutamol every 1–2 hours. They are then weaned accordingly until safely needing only 4–6 puffs every 3–4 hours, at which point they are allowed home. The time taken to reach this point is hugely variable and can last many hours or even days, especially if the exacerbation is related to a viral infection. If the child had no effective treatment prior to your administration of bronchodilators, they may be able to go to four hours between doses very quickly. At the point where discharge is becoming a possibility, ensure that all the criteria for safe discharge (as outlined above in the guideline for mild asthma) are met.

Inhaled bronchodilators are the most important aspect of the acute treatment of any severity of asthma.

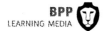

When the severity of an episode is considered 'moderate' it is also time to consider adding systemic steroids. The benefit of bronchodilators is temporary and if large quantities are needed, it is likely that steroids in the form of prednisolone 1–2mg/kg (up to a maximum of 40mg), or equivalent will benefit the child. These doses often alarm those who do not primarily work with children. In the world of paediatrics though, these doses are in common use, and experience shows that they are usually safe. Occasional courses of systemic steroids given for three days seem not to cause harm with any significant regularity. They may however cause the equivalent stimulation of a large coffee.

This side effect should be made known to the parents and, regardless of the timing of the first dose, subsequent doses should be given early in the day for the sake of the parents' sanity.

Once again, improvement should be the norm, so failure to respond to the three 'rescue' doses or deterioration during their administration should prompt reconsideration of the diagnosis. If, as is most likely, the diagnosis remains acute asthma, **failure to respond to treatment is an indication to manage the patient as for a severe, life-threatening episode.**

Flowchart for managing moderate acute asthma

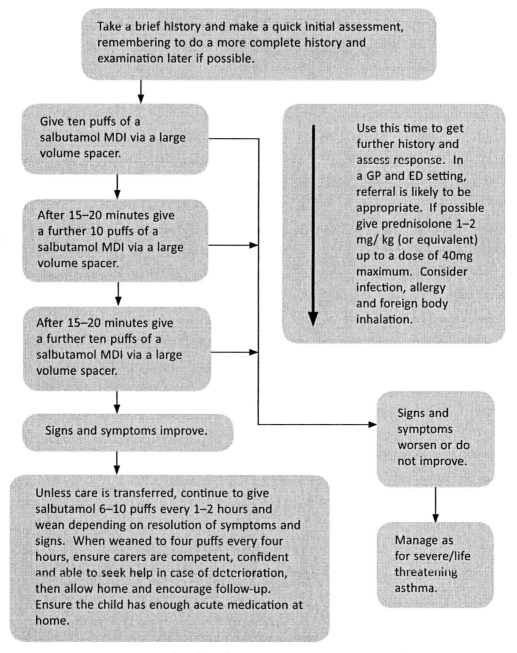

Take a brief history and make a quick initial assessment, remembering to do a more complete history and examination later if possible.

Give ten puffs of a salbutamol MDI via a large volume spacer.

After 15–20 minutes give a further 10 puffs of a salbutamol MDI via a large volume spacer.

After 15–20 minutes give a further ten puffs of a salbutamol MDI via a large volume spacer.

Use this time to get further history and assess response. In a GP and ED setting, referral is likely to be appropriate. If possible give prednisolone 1–2 mg/ kg (or equivalent) up to a dose of 40mg maximum. Consider infection, allergy and foreign body inhalation.

Signs and symptoms improve.

Signs and symptoms worsen or do not improve.

Unless care is transferred, continue to give salbutamol 6–10 puffs every 1–2 hours and wean depending on resolution of symptoms and signs. When weaned to four puffs every four hours, ensure carers are competent, confident and able to seek help in case of deterioration, then allow home and encourage follow-up. Ensure the child has enough acute medication at home.

Manage as for severe/life threatening asthma.

Figure 3.11 Flowchart for managing moderate acute asthma

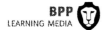

3.4.3 Management of severe/life-threatening acute asthma

Every year, despite aggressive management, a few children die of acute asthma. Make no mistake therefore that **severe asthma is a medical emergency.** There is no role for giving a nebuliser and walking away with the intention of later seeing how well the patient responds. The following are needed order of time:

- **Be calm and reassure the parents and child.** Everyone needs to know that you can see how unwell the child is but at the same time, the confidence that you show will help to avoid unnecessary deterioration due to panicking the child or their parents.
- **Call for help.** In a GP setting, send someone (such as a receptionist) to get an ambulance and get someone else (such as a nurse) to help you with the task of attending to the child. In an emergency department setting, ask for a senior doctor and a nurse who is experienced in treating children to help. Do not accept no for an answer.
- **Assess the airway.** In this circumstance, as long as the child is breathing, and able to physically support themselves, the airway should be considered adequate unless you have cause to believe otherwise. Do not examine the throat unless you have to. You will upset the child and make matters worse.

Do however ask yourself whether the child has wheeze or a stridor or both. (See chapter on stridor and barking cough.)

- **Provide oxygen if you have this available.** Ideally this will be 15 litres/minute via a mask with a reservoir bag at any age.
- **Give a nebuliser of salbutamol if available.** Ideally 5mg over the age of five, and 2.5mg for under-fives. If not available, then give ten puffs of salbutamol via a spacer.
- **Repeat this dose every five minutes** until either the child is taken by ambulance, or a more senior doctor takes over, or the child becomes much better.
- If you get as far as a third nebuliser before someone else takes over care, try to **give an ipratropium nebuliser** alongside the third salbutamol nebuliser. Also **consider giving systemic steroids** if this can be achieved without causing significant upset to the child.

Should the child respond wonderfully to initial treatment, they should still be admitted to a paediatric unit for ongoing observation and treatment. The two most important aspects of ongoing care that you can provide are a dose of systemic steroids and communication with the paediatric team, ensuring that they are under no illusion as to how severely distressed the child was at presentation.

BPP LEARNING MEDIA

Flowchart for managing severe/life-threatening asthma

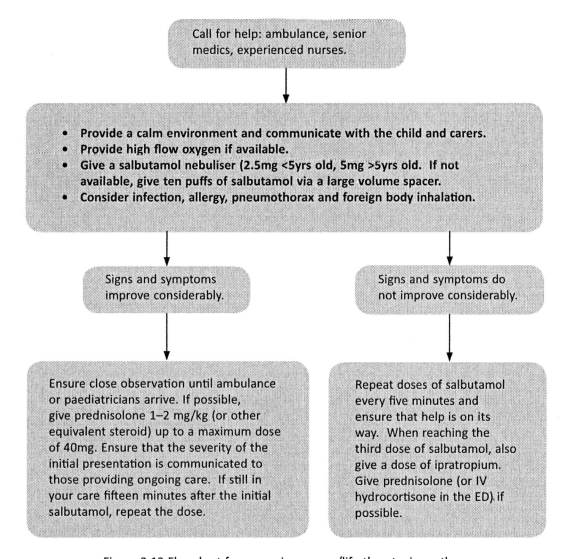

Call for help: ambulance, senior medics, experienced nurses.

- Provide a calm environment and communicate with the child and carers.
- Provide high flow oxygen if available.
- Give a salbutamol nebuliser (2.5mg <5yrs old, 5mg >5yrs old. If not available, give ten puffs of salbutamol via a large volume spacer.
- Consider infection, allergy, pneumothorax and foreign body inhalation.

Signs and symptoms improve considerably.

Signs and symptoms do not improve considerably.

Ensure close observation until ambulance or paediatricians arrive. If possible, give prednisolone 1–2 mg/kg (or other equivalent steroid) up to a maximum dose of 40mg. Ensure that the severity of the initial presentation is communicated to those providing ongoing care. If still in your care fifteen minutes after the initial salbutamol, repeat the dose.

Repeat doses of salbutamol every five minutes and ensure that help is on its way. When reaching the third dose of salbutamol, also give a dose of ipratropium. Give prednisolone (or IV hydrocortisone in the ED) if possible.

Figure 3.12 Flowchart for managing severe/life-threatening asthma

FAQs

Should I use nebulisers or spacers for an acute wheeze?

Wherever possible **the preference should be for using a large volume spacer to initially treat a child who presents with an acute wheeze.**

Nebulisers do have their place but should not be used routinely. As long as you consider the downsides of using a nebuliser and the benefits of using a spacer you should find choosing which to use fairly straightforward.

Nebulised bronchodilators have several disadvantages which are worth knowing:

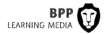

- They are noisy and therefore scary and unwelcome to the child.
- They rely on using much larger amounts of active ingredient. This means that the amount delivered to the lungs is usually enough, but sometimes more than enough and therefore likely to have a systemic effect.
- If the child and parents start to get the idea that nebulisers are better than their own inhalers they may start to rely on medical services to treat exacerbations which they could have managed effectively themselves.
- If a nebuliser is used to treat a wheeze, this is a lost opportunity to see how well the inhaler and spacer are being used at home.
- If a child responds to a nebulised dose of bronchodilator, you have not demonstrated that they are safe to be managed at home.

Using a spacer to treat the child when you see them helps you to be sure that the treatment will continue to be effective after they go home.

Nebulisers are advantageous when you have one of the following situations:

- If you have a completely unco-operative child or there is no one who is able to assist in using the spacer.
- If you need to give facial oxygen at the same time.
- If a child has a severe life-threatening episode.

In these circumstances, I think that nebulisers are your best option.

Summary for acute asthma

- Acute exacerbations of asthma can quickly progress from mild to moderate to life-threatening.
- Early, generous use of bronchodilators is usually very effective.
- Failure to respond to treatment or a need for large doses (>6 puffs of a salbutamol MDI via a large volume spacer) increase the level of concern and should result in escalation of therapy as well as referral to a paediatric unit.
- Anaphylaxis and foreign body aspiration may mimic acute asthma, while pneumothorax may complicate it.

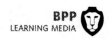

3.4.4 Management of chronic asthma

- Whenever a child presents with an episode of asthma there is an opportunity to improve long term management.
- In order to achieve this you primarily need to remember two words: compliance and avoidance.

Compliance or, as it is now better known, concordance is rarely ideal in the asthmatic child. This is often because the family are used to the child's symptoms and comfortable with the pattern of the child's illness, rather than due to any real neglect. An additional complication is how, as children get older, they prefer to manage their own condition and medication. This, coupled with a desire to be no different from other children, frequently leads to the situation of having children who do not take their inhalers, yet prevent their parent from ensuring that they do so. It is therefore important to establish exactly what is being taken and when.

As most children and carers are keen to believe and convey that they are doing things 'by the book', it is necessary to encourage realism and insist on specifics. In other words, if you ask questions that allow people to give an optimistic view of the way medication is being taken, then an optimistic view is what you are likely to get. In order to encourage realism, it is good

Problem	Solution
The child is having their reliever frequently (more than twice weekly) but not taking a preventer.	Unless this frequent use is for exercise-induced symptoms (which often respond poorly to inhaled steroids) you should encourage the use of, or start, a prophylactic inhaler. Explore any concerns regarding inhaled steroid use. Arrange for follow-up.
The child is using a prophylactic inhaler but too chaotically for this to be effective.	Explain the role of the preventer inhaler. Get the child or carer to incorporate the use of their inhalers into their morning and evening routines. I often suggest that they attach their preventer to their toothbrush by an elastic band so that they remember to use it before brushing their teeth. Try to involve a nurse who has a role in managing chronic asthma.
The child is taking a prophylactic inhaler regularly but their symptoms are still not adequately controlled.	Check technique, then consider dose. Refer to the most up to-date-guidelines such as those from the British Thoracic Society, which can be found in any British National Formulary (BNF). Usually, to 'step up' you need to increase the dose of the steroid inhaler or add in another therapy.
Any smokers In the household	See advice for smokers in the WAVE section (p. 46).
Pets are exacerbating asthma symptoms.	This is always a difficult issue. Although as doctors we want to be seen to have the child's happiness high on our priority list, we also have to be honest about health issues. If the dog (or other pet) is causing the child ill health, then this in turn is probably affecting the child's development and quality of life. You need to be frank that the pet which causes significant morbidity should be removed from the environment.

Figure 3.13 Considering the child's environment as an exacerbating factor

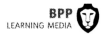

to imply that you do not expect the child to be having their inhalers exactly as prescribed. What you want to know is how the inhalers (or medicines) are being taken. With regard to specifics you want to know how many days a week they remember to take their preventer and how often they need their reliever.

Avoidance of precipitants is equally important. When you have established what is being taken, you should also consider whether the child's environment is an issue. Specifically ask about smoking, pets and whether they think that anything in particular is setting off the child's exacerbations.

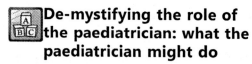

De-mystifying the role of the paediatrician: what the paediatrician might do

The vast majority of children with chronic asthma are managed entirely in primary care. Paediatricians may be involved purely for an acute exacerbation or can share the long term management with the GP. Children who are on high doses of corticosteroids may need to have adrenal function monitored and should be under shared care of a paediatrician.

Summary for chronic asthma

- Chronic asthma is a clinical diagnosis based on the presence of recurrent symptoms such as wheeze, cough and shortness of breath outside of the context of repeated viral respiratory infections. The diagnosis is more likely with a positive family history or the presence of other atopic conditions in the child.
- Although impractical in younger children, from the age of five years peak flow monitoring can be used to support the diagnosis.
- It is rare for children to be taking their inhalers and medicines exactly as prescribed.
- Most chronic asthma can be better controlled by improving compliance, technique and by avoiding precipitants, especially tobacco smoke.
- If needed, increase preventative treatment according to current British Thoracic Society guidelines.
- Good symptom control transforms the lives of the child and parents alike. The aim should be to stop the child from having daily symptoms, although practically it may be impossible to avoid having weekly symptoms.
- Delivering and understanding the medication needed is difficult for parents and child alike. No effort should be spared to provide a practical yet effective preventer and reliever. Regular and opportunistic checks on understanding and concordance are essential.

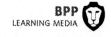

How to be a know-it-all

- Two signs of chronic asthma are mentioned in the overall assessment of the child presenting with an exacerbation of asthma above. Both are caused by the prolonged negative pressure in the thoracic cavity causing deformity of the chest as it grows. One, pectus excavatum, is simply the observation of a sternum which is profoundly depressed toward the spine. This is also a common normal finding but may be a sign of uncontrolled asthma. The second is more specific: Harrison's sulcus is the depression of the lower ribs, creating the appearance of a wide upper chest and a narrowing at the costal margin. This is caused by the continuous pulling of the diaphragm on these lower ribs.

- By contrast, clubbing is not a sign of uncomplicated asthma. Only suppurative lung disease causes clubbing and so, if this phenomenon is found, it should make you consider other or additional diagnoses such as bronchiectasis and cystic fibrosis.

- Although there is no universally accepted definition of asthma, I would offer the following to aid appropriate labelling of children: **asthma is a diagnosis of a chronic tendency to bronchospasm in atopic individuals.** In order to meet the criteria, **a child must have demonstrated their tendency to cough or wheeze over a period of months**, thus excluding those who have a transient cause to their symptoms such as a post-infective cough. Also, to make a confident diagnosis, it is **preferable to have a strong family history** or a past medical history of atopic conditions (eg eczema, asthma, hay fever, true food allergies). Finally, to complete the triad, it is important to be clear that the **symptoms are not occurring solely during times when the child has a cold.** If a child has all three supporting factors, then a more confident diagnosis can be made. When atopy, interval symptoms or definite wheeze are not present then initially it would be preferable to use a non-specific term such as 'possible asthma'. Alternatively simply use a descriptive term such as 'chronic cough' to avoid mislabelling a child when there is diagnostic doubt. Then, when any treatment is given, it will be in the more appropriate context of trialling medication.

- Unlike adults, children have a habit of growing. As a result **children can actually 'grow out of' the dose of steroid inhaler** which they have been started on. Consider this possibility in a previously well-controlled asthmatic child who starts to run into problems.

Also worth knowing

- Not all chronic coughs are symptoms of asthma. One consideration is the possibility that a persistent cough is caused by **pertussis (whooping cough)**. There has been suggestion in recent years that many children have been labelled as asthmatic in their early years when in fact they had the 'one hundred day cough' of pertussis. This can occur in both immunised and non-immunised children, since the vaccine is not 100% protective. Children with pertussis may not present with a classic paroxysmal cough followed by a whoop. Instead they may develop an acute episode without the typical features of whooping cough, which then settles down into a nuisance cough. By the time that the child's parents have sought medical advice for the nth time it is understandable

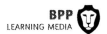

that the doctor consulted would be desperately searching for a possible treatment. However since the natural history of this condition is to resolve after a few months, the impression will be that anything prescribed, such as a steroid inhaler, was responsible for resolving the symptoms. For this reason, it is worth considering holding off from treating a 'nuisance cough' (ie a dry cough which seems to be affecting the parents, while the child is thriving, well and unperturbed) for the first few months. This is especially true the younger the child is, since in these patients true chronic wheeze is less likely and pertussis is more common.

- Another cause of cough that fails to improve is **foreign body inhalation**. Children have a nasty habit of inhaling things and after the initial choking episode the child may be reassuringly well. However in any child who has a nuisance cough, or recurrent lower respiratory tract infections the possibility of a foreign body lodged in a bronchus must be considered. Look for persistent collapse or air trapping on an X-ray.

- Although not universally accepted as a condition, many experts will tell you that **chronic endo-bronchial infection** is an under-diagnosed cause for chronic cough in children. This is thought to be a low-grade chronic infection of the bronchial endothelium which may be a precursor to bronchiectasis. The clue that a child may have this condition comes from the pattern of illness. They often have a ruttly, wet cough for many weeks, which resolves temporarily or partially improves when antibiotics are given. If a child follows this pattern of symptoms, then chronic endobronchial infection may be the reason for not improving. Because these infections are in the bronchi rather than the alveoli,

the infection is more difficult to treat. It is reasonable to give children with this clinical picture four weeks of co-amoxiclav. If they get better and do not relapse, there is no obligation to refer.

- Streptococcal pneumonia (the most common bacterial cause of pneumonia in children) causes lower respiratory tract infections that are not usually complicated by wheeze. If therefore, a child develops first a cough and then a wheeze, and a lower respiratory tract infection is diagnosed, the likelihood is that the infection is viral or atypical bacterial pneumonia. Mycoplasma infection, for example, does commonly cause wheeze.

- However, if an episode of asthma is complicated subsequently by a bacterial infection, then common or garden Streptococcal pneumonia should be top of your list of suspects. In theory, noting the sequence of events should therefore help to determine the first choice antibiotic when treating infection in the setting of wheezy episodes.

FAQs

What is the best inhaler for children?

The short answer to this is that **the best device for any child is the one that they can and will use, with two notable exceptions (salbutamol syrup and nebulisers, explained below).** Realism is important in choosing a device for a child. The best delivery (maximum delivery to the bronchial tree, minimal delivery to the pharynx and the least systemic absorption) remains via an aerosol MDI, given with good technique via a large volume spacer. However, even with experienced patients and parents, technique is rarely good and many are reluctant to carry a large spacer around with them. Because of this reason, there are many devices that are compact and most are effective and easy to use. In order to determine which device is best for a

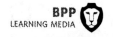

child you need to consider their age and their circumstances. Ultimately, what you really want is a nurse who has demonstration devices and the time to go through them so that a usable device can be selected.

Notable exception number one is salbutamol syrup. It is my opinion that **there is now no longer a place for the use of salbutamol syrup** as a way of giving β-agonist when needed acutely, for the following reasons:

- It relies on systemic absorption, delaying the effect dramatically.
- Due to this mechanism of action, via the systemic route, it needs to be given in doses that are ten or more times greater than the effective inhaled dose. This causes significant side effects. I have often heard parents tell me how their children have been tremulous after just one spoonful.
- There is no age group of children who are unable to use an MDI with spacer. The available range of spacers and masks is excellent. Therefore there is no cohort of children who can 'only take syrup'.

The second delivery method which should be avoided outside the hospital setting is the use of nebulisers. The reason for this is that there is a real risk that a child will be at home, having a nebuliser for an acute attack, and the nebuliser will mask the severity of the episode. When the child deteriorates, this may happen dramatically. Again, the MDI with spacer is a good, effective and versatile method of initially treating any episode. It allows the child to have small doses, and if they don't respond to this, it can be used to deliver increased doses. However it will be noted that they needed the increased dose, and help can be sought.

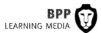**What do I tell the parents?**

When a child is having an exacerbation of asthma that can be managed initially at home:

"Because giving a larger number of puffs of your child's usual inhaler has settled their wheeze and breathing down so much, I think that it is possible to let you go home. Children who get dangerous episodes of asthma are usually the ones who get a good dose of inhalers and don't really get much better. (Because your child has started on steroid medicine, I would hope that this will also make it more likely that they will improve rather than get worse.) At home, you should give 4-6 puffs of the blue inhaler through the plastic bubble every 3–4 hours. If your child gets worse sooner than that or doesn't improve with the inhalers, you should get seen again. You may need to do this for a day or two but you should also see a general improvement. If things are getting worse, it is better to get seen earlier than later."

"Because your child is well aside from the wheeze and difficulty breathing, I don't think antibiotics will help. However if your child developed a fever or was unwell in themselves, that would be another reason to get them checked over again."

When I want to advise about managing chronic asthma:

"Perfecting the treatment of asthma is not easy. It can be very difficult to remember to give medicines and inhalers every day, especially if your child seems fine or is just used to having their cough and wheeze. It is important to be sure about which inhaler does what and when they should be used, because it must be confusing at times. Treatment gets changed so often, and different people are always telling you different things. That is why it is best to see someone regularly who knows you and whom you trust, such as a GP or asthma nurse. Make sure that they are providing you with medicines and inhalers that you can give easily. You should also make sure that if you have any problems or don't understand anything you ask questions whenever you can."

"There are two kinds of treatments for asthma, relievers and preventers. Both are very important. Relievers need to be given every time your child has a wheeze or feels short of breath. Sometimes a cough can also be a sign that the tubes in the chest are tight.

Giving a reliever quickly is a good way of making it less likely that your child will get a bad episode."

"Because relievers do usually work so well it is easy to find yourself using those and forgetting to give the preventer treatment. However, the preventers are usually very effective if you remember to take them every day. By doing this your child will feel better in themselves, sleep better and feel able to do more things."

"Sometimes it is also possible to find other ways of making asthma a bit better. If a smoker lives inside the house, this is a big cause of asthma. Smoking outside is better than smoking inside, but really stopping smoking is the only effective way to stop the cigarette smoke on your clothes and in your breath from triggering asthma symptoms. Another thing that some people find useful is getting a new pillow every few months. This is because there are bugs too tiny to see that eat dead skin and live in the pillows. Getting rid of old pillows reduces the amount that you child breathes in these bugs that set off asthma."

Summary for asthma

- Respiratory illness is the most common reason for children to present for acute medical assessment.
- Most children will have an uncomplicated viral upper respiratory tract infection. Such cases are best managed with over-the-counter remedies. Antibiotics and steroids are not indicated unless there is a clear indication.
- Children with wheeze and/or respiratory distress are likely to have bronchiolitis, a wheeze associated viral episode or asthma. By making one of these diagnoses it is possible to direct the appropriate treatment to the child.
- Most wheezing children can be managed in the community; however, all of the above conditions can be progressive and life-threatening. Early escalation of treatment should be considered when a child is more unwell, or has respiratory distress or fails to respond to initial treatment.

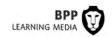

Chapter 4

The child with stridor and/or a barking cough

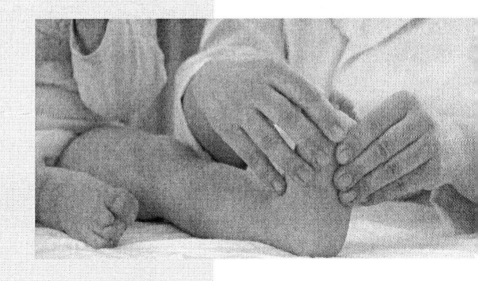

The child with stridor and/or a barking cough

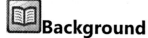

Background

- Stridor and a barking cough are both signs of a narrowing of the upper airway.
- Stridor can be difficult to recognise, and may easily be mistaken for wheeze.
- It is important to recognise the difference because the causes and treatment of stridor are different to that of acute wheeze.
- Stridor has many possible causes, each affecting different age groups. Some causes are common and others are rare. Knowing what the possible causes are and the way that they present will lead to a speedy diagnosis in most cases.

The most important step is deciding that the child has a stridor. To begin with then, the child needs to have noisy breathing. Sometimes this can be quite subtle but, unlike wheeze, a subtle stridor is usually an early stridor (remember that wheezes often get quieter as air entry diminishes and the child deteriorates), so a quiet noise is reassuring unless the child has an altered consciousness. If it is an obvious noise, then determining whether it is a wheeze or a stridor is easier. In this case the timing and the character of the noise will help to determine which of these two phenomena you are hearing.

Because the upper airways are opened by air pushing through them in expiration. and relatively collapsed when air is sucked through in inspiration, stridor is predominantly a noise of inspiration. Therefore, if the noise accompanies chest expansion or intercostal recession (ie the noise occurs in inspiration) then you should call it a stridor.

A wheeze follows the opposite pattern and is predominantly a noise of expiration. However,

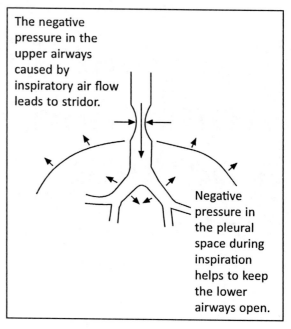

The negative pressure in the upper airways caused by inspiratory air flow leads to stridor.

Negative pressure in the pleural space during inspiration helps to keep the lower airways open.

Figure 4.1 The physics of stridor

note that both wheeze and stridor can occur in inspiration and expiration because the constriction narrows, causing turbulence to occur when air is flowing in either direction.

The character of the sound is also helpful in deciding what you are dealing with. While a wheeze is a whistling sound, stridor is a rasping sound. The notable exception to this is the baby with stridor. When they have a stridor, these tiny tots make a sound which can only be described as a squeak. If you ever hear one, you will be struck by the oddness of the sound.

A barking cough is just what it says it is. It sounds unmistakably like a seal or a dog barking. This sound is similarly created by collapse of the upper airway during expiration. It may be present along with a stridor or it may occur on its own and later possibly progress to a stridor.

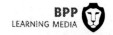

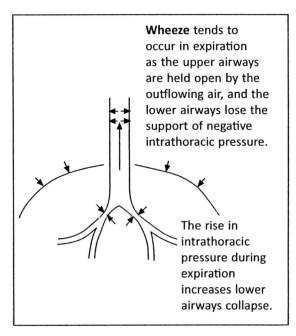

Wheeze tends to occur in expiration as the upper airways are held open by the outflowing air, and the lower airways lose the support of negative intrathoracic pressure.

The rise in intrathoracic pressure during expiration increases lower airways collapse.

Figure 4.2 The physics of wheeze

How to assess

If a child presents with stridor or a barking cough then they have an airway problem. In assessing your patient you therefore have two main tasks:

1. **Assess quickly.**
2. **Do not upset your patient.**

Therefore this is one situation where the more that you assess from a distance, the better the outcome is likely to be. So without upsetting the child, assess the following:

- Is the child in respiratory distress? Assess the work and efficacy of breathing.
- **If the child is distressed or hypoxic, give facial oxygen where available as long as this does not upset the child too much.**

- If the child looks unwell or is working moderately hard, then call for help now.
- If the child is extremely well and tolerating the examination, take a full history and do a full examination.
- Ask about the onset of symptoms. What started this off? How quickly have they become this bad?
- Have there been any choking episodes, especially at meal times or play times?
- Has the child had this problem before and how bad has it been at its worst?
- Has the child ever had endotracheal intubation? Have they had any operations? Have they been on the special care baby unit (SCBU) as a baby?
- If possible, examine the child in the order of what you most want to determine, but be prepared to stop if you make the child cry, or the stridor becomes worse. Look especially for the following:
  - Listen to the chest for air entry and to assess whether there is also a wheeze and therefore a lower respiratory component.
  - Palpate for lymph nodes in the neck, as a way of assessing whether there might be infection.
  - Assess the circulation. What is the pulse? What is the capillary refill time? What are the heart sounds like?
- Note that the throat is not on the list of things to examine. **You must not examine the throat, as this can cause a sudden deterioration** by precipitating further swelling as you stretch the soft tissues of the neck.

The information that you have gathered will now almost certainly allow you to make a diagnosis based on one of the following patterns of signs and symptoms.

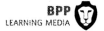

Condition	Typical age at onset	Signs and symptoms
Laryngomalacia	From shortly after birth to one year	Squeaking stridor. Often intermittent and with a non-acute onset. May have been present from shortly after birth but not usually at birth. Not usually associated with a cough. May suddenly get worse during times of upper respiratory tract infection. Otherwise w child. These children usually do not look distressed when they present.
Sub-glottic stenosis	From birth onwards	This is a narrowing of the trachea due to scar tissue. There is almost always a past history of endotracheal intubation, though the stridor often occurs well after the initial trauma. The stridor may be intermittent and may be worsened during times of upper respiratory tract infection. Usually a well child with no worrying findings on examination.
Foreign body inhalation	From the age when the child can crawl (may be earlier if siblings are giving small objects to them)	Sudden onset of stridor, without fever or systemic illness. There may or may not be a history of choking. If there *is* a possible episode, then it will usually be very recent-you cannot tolerate a foreign body in your upper airway or trapped in your oesophagus for long. Note that if the foreign body moves into the lower airways, it will produce a wheeze or cough, not a stridor. It is also possible for foreign bodies to remain undetected for much longer once they are intrathoracic.
Croup	Usually over one year of age	Tends to start with a characteristic and impressive barking cough before usually, but not always, progressing to stridor. There is often a coryza which precedes the onset. The degree of respiratory distress is very variable but very important. It is often the case that the child has had previous episodes of croup.
Epiglottitis and bacterial tracheitis	Rare in any age group	These children are usually severely unwell. The non-immunised child should be considered most at risk of these deadly infections. Typically the child will look very ill and sit forward, drooling forth the saliva which they cannot swallow due to the painful swelling in the laryngo-pharynx. They have fevers, are systemically unwell and become more unwell by the minute. Although they are septic, it is the rapid worsening of the upper airway that is most dramatic. **A stridor in an unwell child is due to bacterial infection until proved otherwise.**

Figure 4.3 Patterns of signs and symptoms for diagnosis.

The 'must do's

- ☑ **If there is respiratory distress, the child with barking cough or stridor must be managed as a medical emergency.**
- ☑ If stridor is suspected, but wheeze also seems to be present, then it is reasonable to treat as for both problems.
- ☑ If the child looks well, then fully assess the story and the child.
- ☑ If the child is unwell, then call for urgent help and start simple measures such as providing oxygen and a calm environment.

Pitfalls to avoid

- ☒ **Never examine the child's throat.** Any disturbance of the upper airways can worsen the narrowing and lead to collapse.
- ☒ **Never do anything painful to the child.** If they need intravenous access because they are so unwell, this must wait until they are somewhere with an anaesthetist and hopefully also an ENT surgeon. It is better to allow them to have some cardiovascular compromise than complete airway obstruction.

How to be a know-it-all

Laryngomalacia and tracheomalacia are conditions that usually present in small babies. They occur due to inadequate cartilage being present to support the upper airways. This floppiness is present to some degree in all newborns, and as stronger cartilage usually develops, these problems tend to resolve as the child grows. This improvement occurs because the airways become larger and more rigid cartilage develops in time.

Recognising these conditions provides a delightful opportunity to be able to give the anxious parent a 'this is almost certainly a floppy breathing tube' diagnosis after simply taking a history and examining the child. The 'squeak' that these babies produce is unmistakeable. It will be apparent that the child is well and the history will usually identify a reassuringly intermittent and non-acute onset. It is important to consider the possibility that the child has been intubated at birth (sub-glottic stenosis is a differential in these children) but the parent will usually know if this was the case. Neonatal resuscitation no longer favours suctioning of the vocal cords, and it is rare to intubate a newborn compared to past paediatric practices. More importantly, sub-glottic stenosis usually results from prolonged intubation. So apart from rare anatomical abnormalities (vascular rings, etc), when you see a baby which has a longstanding stridor with no ill effect, you can confidently tell the parents that their child has a 'floppy windpipe'.

Even if you don't hear the squeak yourself, the parents may describe what is happening well enough to make the diagnosis. You will now be even more so the hero. It is often the case that the poor parents have been noticing this noise for some time but that the child has been frustratingly silent whenever they go near a doctor or health visitor. Again, it is reasonable to give a confident diagnosis if the history strongly suggests laryngomalacia. You can then choose to monitor them yourself or refer to an ENT specialist to confirm the diagnosis (see below).

Stridor that presents at birth or within hours of birth should be considered significant pathology even in the absence of distress. These children are less likely to have laryngomalacia and should be discussed with a specialist.

Finally, there is an association between capillary haemangiomas (strawberry naevi) on the face and laryngeal haemangiomas. If a child with a strawberry naevus had a squeak then I would suggest phoning an ENT surgeon in these cases as well.

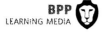

Also worth knowing

Laryngomalacia is associated with gastro-oesophageal reflux for two reasons.

1. Babies with laryngomalacia develop reflux more often, either because they need greater negative intrathoracic pressures to breathe (which encourage milk to move up the oesophagus) or perhaps because one floppy bit here is associated with another floppy valve elsewhere.

2. Reflux causes inflammation, so a swollen epiglottis may worsen any narrowing due to floppiness that is already there. It is therefore worth looking for evidence of reflux and treating it if it is there in these babies.

Managing problems with the upper airways

Condition	Suggested management
Tracheomalacia, laryngomalacia, and sub-glottic stenosis	In the past, it was normal practice to follow all these babies up without investigating them if they were well and thriving. However flexible laryngoscopy (without need for a general anaesthetic) has made it possible for ENT surgeons to more easily assess these children. The benefit of getting such an assessment is to rule out rarer causes such as vocal cord immobility. If you were to monitor a presumed laryngomalacia without referring them, only do so if the child is thriving, not having choking episodes, frequent infections, apnoeas or reflux.
Foreign body inhaled or swallowed	If suspected, then arrange for urgent assessment by an ENT surgeon. If the child is comfortable in a particular position, allow them to remain in that position. Minimal movement will allow them to protect their own airway in most cases.
Croup	See flowchart below. Note that croup is a viral infection, and so antibiotics are not indicated.
Epiglottitis and bacterial tracheitis	As soon as this is suspected, the child needs to be taken to the nearest resuscitation room available. An anaesthetist and an ENT surgeon should be present as soon as is possible, at which point the child needs their airway securing however necessary. At the same time the child can be given oxygen, intravenous antibiotics and fluids.

Figure 4.4 Managing problems with the upper airways

De-mystifying the role of the paediatrician: what the paediatrician might do

- The majority of children with barking coughs are managed in general practice or the emergency department. This is because in most cases there is a cough and no stridor or significant respiratory distress.
- In the emergency department or a general practice setting where a period of observation is available, it is possible to manage moderate episodes by treating and seeing whether the child improves or deteriorates.

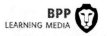

- The main role of the paediatrician is to be involved in the less straightforward cases and the more severe cases.
- For the atypical children (ex-premature babies, babies with minor heart defects, adverse social circumstances etc) the paediatrician will simply admit to observe rather than have a child outside of hospital who could deteriorate rapidly.
- For the severe cases the paediatrician will escalate treatment and will occasionally need to be part of the pathway to admitting the child to a paediatric intensive care unit.

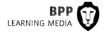What do I tell the parents?

When I am sending home a child who has croup:

"Your child has croup. This is a viral infection of the voice box which is quite common in young children. Sometimes it is very mild and doesn't need any treatment and other times it is a bit more of a nuisance, which is when we tend to use steroid medicines to reduce the swelling which is the cause of the difficulties.

Sometimes it can become a severe tightening of the tubes. When this is the case, children need to be in hospital for their treatment."

"Because your child is doing well with their breathing at the moment I am happy to let you take your child home. However if their breathing becomes worse or noisy, or you feel that there is something else you are unhappy about, you should bring them back. I think that they are very likely going to be fine but if they seem to become worse quickly, you should phone an ambulance."

"Nothing that you can do at home will really make any difference to what happens next. Some people recommend making steam but this is not proven to help. The only important thing is to make sure that they stay away from tobacco smoke and anyone who has been smoking. The cough itself will be there for another couple of days. It takes a different amount of time to go in every child but you should find that no matter how long it takes, it does generally get better each day. You might also find that the croupy cough returns with the next cold that your child catches. If the cough does come back, then unless you are completely happy with your child, you should get them assessed again. No one will think that you are being an anxious parent."

Flowchart for assessing and treating the child with croup

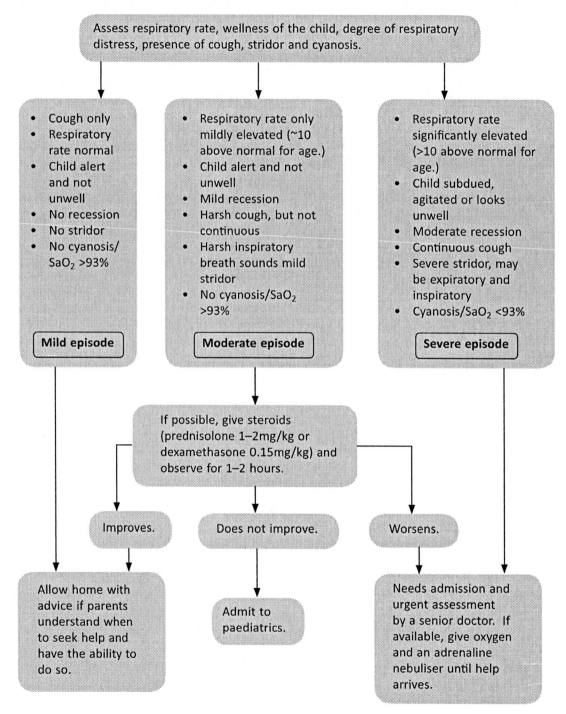

Figure 4.5 Flowchart for assessing and treating the child with croup

Summary for the child with stridor and/or a barking cough

- Stridor usually sounds harsh and rasping and occurs mainly in inspiration.
- Stridor and barking cough are indicators of partial upper airways obstruction.
- Loss of airway leads more rapidly to death than lower respiratory failure or cardiovascular collapse.
- The cause can usually be identified from the history and clinical assessment.
- Although there are several possible causes of stridor and barking cough, the most common cause in childhood is croup.
- Although most cases of croup are mild and require no treatment, or moderate and respond well to steroids, care must be taken to identify the cases of severe or worsening croup as these can be life threatening.

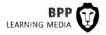

Chapter 5

The febrile or unsettled child with non-specific symptoms

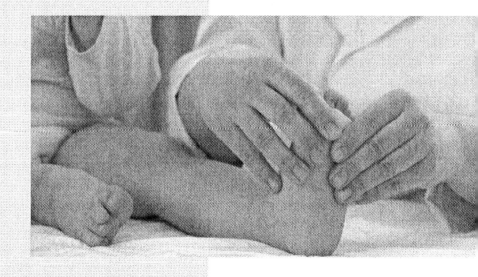

The febrile or unsettled child with non-specific symptoms

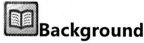**Background**

The chances are, if you are using this text as a reference book rather than going from cover to cover, that you may have come to this chapter first. Children often present with a fever and a parent or carer looks to you for answers. You may or may not be able to find a cause but if you do then this will help you to reassure that parent about their child's symptoms.

Your agenda should be to:

- Try to find a cause that you can treat.
- Exclude possible serious explanations for the child's symptoms.
- Provide an explanation of the symptoms or, if you find none, refer where appropriate.
- Recognise that you are only able to assess the child as they are. Some children who have minor infections later develop serious infections, so safety-netting well and arranging observation where appropriate are vital.

This may seem a challenge in the context of a busy emergency department and virtually impossible in the context of a general practice consultation. However the odds are in fact on your side. Most of these children do not have serious infections. Furthermore, if you listen to the warnings you will most likely recognise the child with more significant illness.

This group of patients constitute a significant chunk of children who present to primary care. The aim should be to manage the vast majority of them in primary care, since unnecessary referral causes considerable anxiety and inconvenience.

How to assess

- Ask about what symptoms the child has, when the symptoms started and whether the symptoms are getting better, worse or staying the same.
- Ask about contact with any infections and letters which have come home from school about outbreaks of contagious illnesses.
- Try to assess how ill the child is by asking:
  - How ill do the parents feel their child is?
  - Does the child seem like their normal self? If not, then how are they different?
  - What is the child is doing and not doing that they normally do? Playing and eating are children's favourite pastimes so if these activities have stopped, you should see that as significant.
- Ask about fevers and ask for specific numbers if they have taken their temperature.
- Ask specifically about coughs, diarrhoea, vomiting, pain and urinary symptoms.
- Examine the child fully.
- **It is essential to gain a good look at both of the ear drums as well as the pharynx** (not just the palate) in order to confidently diagnose or rule out an upper respiratory tract infection (URTI). If you haven't seen tonsils and ear drums, then you haven't finished examining the child.
- Even if an URTI is found, this does not exclude other concurrent and possibly related illnesses. It is still therefore important to examine the heart, lungs, abdomen and make a neurological assessment.
- Look for a rash. Ideally, this means full exposure of the child.
- **Unless a clear focus for infection is found, obtain a urine specimen for testing.**

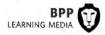

In fact, have a low threshold for doing this whenever in doubt. Though inconvenient to obtain, it is a harmless test, and urine infections can be easily missed.

Your assessment will give you the underlying cause in the majority of cases. The likely diagnosis will depend on the age of the child, and their symptoms and signs. Below are tables to aid decision-making. These tables are based on the age of the child, as the likelihood of different conditions and the way that each condition presents alters with each stage of childhood.

> If the tonsils are visualised, this is the indication that an adequate view of a child's throat has been achieved.

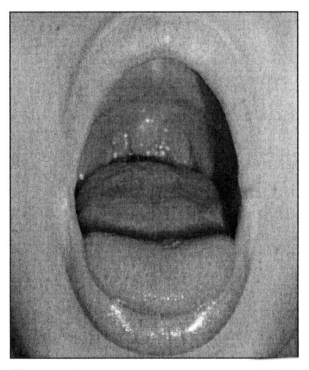

Figure 5.1 Throat examination of a 13-year-old child

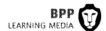

From birth to six months

Possible condition	Characteristics, symptoms and signs
Upper respiratory tract infection (URTI)	• Coryzal, or inflamed pharynx or ear drums. • No signs of sepsis. • Be very hesitant to diagnose this in children under three months old if febrile.
Lower respiratory tract infection (LRTI)	• Uncommon at this age. • Usually has cough and respiratory distress – these accompanying a significant fever equal a LRTI unless proven otherwise. • Auscultation signs are variable and unreliable. There can be crepitations with no infection and an infection with no crepitations.
Urinary tract infection (UTI)	• Presents with unsettled babies, who may or may not be unwell. • Have a very low threshold for excluding UTI in this age group, as sepsis can develop rapidly. • There are usually no specific signs and the absence of an explanation of a fever or for an unsettled child should make the exclusion of UTI mandatory.
Meningitis	• Presents with very unsettled babies. • Classically they have a high pitched 'irritable' cry. • Instead of neck stiffness, these babies have increased tone and do not respond kindly to being handled. • There may be a bulging fontanelle, even when not crying. • Although classically associated with sepsis, meningitis may precede sepsis.
Sepsis (which may be due to any of the above)	• Presents as an unwell baby but not always dramatically so. The baby may just seem 'not their normal self' or be 'off their feeds'. • Usually, either the parent, the doctor or the nurse get a sense of foreboding about a child with sepsis. • Suspect sepsis if heart rate is high, capillary refill is prolonged or the baby is subdued. • Pure sepsis may present without a focal infection. As a result, absence of a good explanation for a baby's unwellness leaves developing sepsis as a possibility. In other words, the child with fever who is unwell and has no focal findings is presumed to be septic.

Figure 5.2 Characteristics, symptoms and signs from birth to six months

Six months to three years

Possible condition	Characteristics, symptoms and signs
Upper respiratory tract infection (URTI)	• Extremely common in this age group, especially if at nursery or has older siblings in which case URTIs may occur more than once a month. • Coryza I, or inflamed pharynx or ear drums. • No signs of sepsis in uncomplicated URTI. If the child is significantly unwell, consider concurrent or complicating infections.
Lower respiratory tract infection (LRTI)	• More common at this age but if present is usually viral. • Usually has cough and respiratory distress – these accompanying a significant fever equal a LRTI unless proven otherwise. • Auscultation signs are variable and unreliable. There can be crepitations with no infection and an infection with no crepitations.
Urinary tract infection (UTI)	• Presents with miserable children, who may or may not be unwell. • There are usually no specific signs and the absence of a focus for infection should make the exclusion of UTI mandatory.
Meningitis	• Presents with irritable children. • Suspect meningitis in the subdued child who will not settle. • Neck stiffness or increased tone may be present. • Although classically associated with sepsis, meningitis may precede sepsis.
Sepsis (which may be due to any of the above)	• This will be a noticeably unwell child. • Usually, either the parent, the doctor or the nurse get a sense of foreboding about a child with sepsis. • Suspect sepsis if heart rate is high, capillary refill is prolonged or the child is subdued. • Assume that sepsis is present when a child is unwell and no focus can be found. • May be accompanied by a progressive petechial or purpuric rash.

Figure 5.3 Characteristics, symptoms and signs from six months to three years

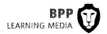

Three years to adulthood

Possible condition	Characteristics, symptoms and signs
Upper respiratory tract infection (URTI)	• Continues to be the most common cause of fever. • Coryzal, or inflamed pharynx or ear drums. May also now complain of specific symptoms such as earache or sore throat. • If signs of sepsis, then this is evidence of systemic bacterial infection in addition to the URTI.
Lower respiratory tract infection (LRTI)	• Bacterial infections become increasingly common in the older child. • Usually has a cough and respiratory distress – these accompanying a significant fever equal a LRTI unless proven otherwise. • Auscultation signs are variable and unreliable. There can be crepitations with no infection and an infection with no crepitations.
Urinary tract infection (UTI)	• Presents with vague abdominal pains. Sometimes also age-appropriate urinary symptoms: enuresis in the younger child and frequency/dysuria in the older child • There are still usually no specific signs. • Tenderness in the renal angles suggests kidney involvement.
Meningitis	• Presents with headache, photophobia or just being quite unwell. • Suspect meningitis in the subdued child who does not seem their normal self. • Neck stiffness or increased tone may be present. By this age, it is possible to test for Kernig's sign.
Sepsis (which may be due to any of the above)	• This will be a noticeably unwell child. • Usually, either the parent, the doctor or the nurse get a sense of foreboding about a child with sepsis. • Suspect sepsis if heart rate is high, capillary refill is prolonged or the child is subdued. • Assume that sepsis is present when a child is unwell and no focus can be found. • May be accompanied by a progressive petechial or purpuric rash.

Figure 5.4 Characteristics, symptoms and signs from three years to adulthood

The 'must do's

- ☑ **Significant effort spent on gaining a good look at both ear drums and the pharynx is time well spent**. Unless the child is able to cooperate (and many children do surprisingly well at this), you require an adult who is willing to hold the child tight no matter how much they fight. Then to complete your side of the bargain you need to look swiftly, yet accurately. Firm but gentle is the way to gain a good view humanely. Remember though that being too gentle is no good to anyone. The likelihood is that the child who is going to get upset will be upset regardless, so make sure that you make a good effort and don't be too put off by a child who doesn't want to be examined. If the child is really too combative and the adult isn't managing to hold the child still, you may need to stop, suggest that another adult tries holding the child and show them exactly how to do so again, before having another attempt. Giving up without obtaining a view should not be necessary.
- ☑ Listen to the parents' anxieties. If you have made an assessment and explained your findings then **it is part of the safe completion of your consultation to ask the parents if they still have any worries**. If they do, then it may be because there is something wrong with the child that they have been unable to articulate or you did not fully appreciate. If you cannot reassure the parents, do not be too quick to dismiss these anxieties.
- ☑ You should **take high temperatures (>39°C) seriously** but in the context of the whole child. Septic children do not usually look well. In other words, a cheerful child with a high temperature is less likely to have a serious illness than a miserable or very subdued child with the same temperature. However you should feel more obliged to justify your opinion that the child is well the higher the temperature is that is recorded.
- ☑ Likewise any 'fever effects' should be taken seriously. A rigor potentially implies a more serious infection. While it is possible for a child with a simple viral infection to have a conscious shaking episode, the presence of a rigor in the history should make any clinician more wary, have a lower threshold to investigate and more keen to observe the child.

Pitfalls to avoid

- ☒ Mastoiditis is easy to miss. This is because it may be hidden by hair or the ear and so needs examining for specifically. Have a look at the child's face and ask yourself if one of the ears is pushed forwards. Then look for redness and swelling behind the ears. Finally, at the same time as you examine for lymph nodes in the neck, palpate the mastoid bone behind the ear. It may be tender or there may be a boggy swelling.

How to be a know-it-all

The majority of children with febrile illnesses have one of the common (or less common but more serious) infections listed above. There are however a few children who present with fevers who have less common causes. While it is unnecessary to know these conditions in detail, knowing how to spot them is extremely valuable. A child who presents without a straightforward history and examination should have the following problems considered.

- **Complications of bacterial upper respiratory tract infection** are thankfully rare but do occur and catch out the unwary clinician. **Peritonsillar abscesses ('quinsy'), mastoiditis and brain abscesses** are three such invasive

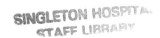

infections. These will usually make the child more unwell and may present with specific symptoms (unable to swallow in quinsy, neurological symptoms in brain abscesses) or signs (see pitfalls). However note that children who have recently had an oral broad spectrum antibiotic may have these conditions partially treated. It is useful in such children to examine them more thoroughly, than for a child presenting at the beginning of an illness and who has been well for the preceding few weeks. If there are signs or symptoms that a recent infection has become invasive, refer.

- **Septic arthritis** will usually present with localising symptoms in older children. However in preverbal children or if no focus has been found, the only way to rule an infected joint out as the source of the fever is to examine arms and legs. The simplest way to do this is to get the child to use their limbs and be confident that there is no restriction. A child will not allow movement of an infected joint.

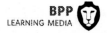

Also worth knowing

Kawasaki's disease has many of the features of a viral illness but is an important diagnosis to make because early treatment may reduce cardiac complications. Important features to look for are:

- A really miserable child. Children with viral illnesses are often miserable but settle with medication and there is a steady improvement over the space of a few days. Children with Kawasaki's are more consistently and persistently miserable.
- There will be a fever that persists for five days and does not improve with antibiotic treatment.
- Most will have conjunctivitis but no discharge.
- Most will have a non-specific rash.
- Most will have inflammation of the oral mucosa.

- About half will have lymphadenopathy which will be more dramatic than that expected for a viral URTI.
- While peeling skin on hands and feet are the sign that most people associate with Kawasaki's, it is a late occurrence and not always present.

Children who continue to be febrile five days into an infection that was originally felt to be viral are still more likely to have a bacterial infection, so all the possibilities must be considered. However, children with a fever for five days and who fulfil the diagnostic criteria should be referred as soon as the diagnosis is significant possibility.

General management of the febrile or unsettled child

Temperature control

There are two aspects to managing these children. While treatment of the underlying infection is important (where it is possible), the second goal is the treatment of the pain and fever associated with the infection. Fever control is important to help the child feel better and to give you a true picture of how unwell the child is. Treating a high temperature and the associated misery is achieved both through medication and other means. In order to achieve maximum temperature control, consider the following:

- **Is the child able to shed heat?** Children are often wrapped up very warmly to come to be seen by the doctor. They should be stripped down to a minimum of clothing as long as the room temperature is not cold. Don't overdo this though. Cold air and fans, like sponging, can cause vasoconstriction and cause the core temperature to paradoxically rise. If the skin is cooled too much the child may shiver which will also raise core temperature.

- **Has the child been receiving antipyretics at home?** If so, how much? Parents often hold back for a variety of reasons. They do not want to 'fill their children with too many medicines' and many over the counter medicines advise that they are not to be given for more than three days without consulting a physician.

The management of fever is therefore best achieved by ensuring that the child is adequately exposed and that they have received the maximum allowed dose (according to weight or age) of at least one antipyretic medication.

Specific management of the febrile or unsettled child

The management of each condition depends on what it is. URTI has been covered already in Chapter 3. The following sections outline an approach to the other conditions that may be encountered.

5.1 Lower respiratory tract infection (LRTI)

Assessment

As mentioned previously, diagnosing LRTI is far from straightforward. **Most children with a cough and crackles heard on auscultation do not have a LRTI.** Also, many children with LRTI do not have obvious signs in the chest. Because of this difficulty many doctors develop a policy of treating with antibiotics whenever a LRTI *might* be present. Unfortunately this means that any child with a cough is treated with antibiotics, and the vast majority of these children are being put at risk of antibiotic side effects unnecessarily.

Note that the term 'lower respiratory tract infection' essentially means any infection of the respiratory system within the thoracic cavity. This could mean a viral or bacterial infection and could mean bronchitis or pneumonia. I have intentionally used the rather vague LRTI to reflect the uncertainty that we all have as doctors when making the diagnosis of a 'chest infection'. However, with a child who has focal signs and is clearly unwell and in distress, the term pneumonia is obviously more medically appropriate.

My approach to diagnosing LRTI is one which I think allows the clinician to treat 'in case' where appropriate but is likely to ensure as accurate a 'hit rate' as possible in this tricky condition. I believe that a healthy mix of suspicion and scepticism are needed to assess children regarding the possibility of LRTI.

Of course, the child as a whole needs to be the factor that truly makes your mind up regarding the diagnosis. However, I think that 'unpacking' the various factors and considering how much weight to give them is important. The following is a guide to the factors which may help to make a diagnosis, according to how significant I think that they are:

Unlike in adult medicine, blood tests and chest X-rays are not a routine part of diagnosing or managing pneumonia in children. Irradiating children should be avoided unless truly needed and should never be done 'routinely'. Children are vulnerable and the benefits of a test should be clear before a child is subjected to the distress associated with venepuncture. In general, blood tests and X-rays should not be needed to diagnose LRTI and may even confuse the diagnosis as changes lag after clinical signs of infection. Investigations do have a role but mainly in the management of LRTI severe enough to require admission to hospital. Therefore as a rule, investigations should not be needed to make a decision to refer to the paediatric team.

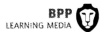

Signs that are significant and suggest possible LRTI	Signs which may suggest LRTI	Signs which are non specific for LRTI
• Respiratory distress without wheeze • Focal reduced breath sounds on auscultation • Localised dullness to percussion • Localised bronchial breathing on auscultation	• Focal crepitations on auscultation • Fever • Unwell child	• Cough, even if productive • Scattered crepitations on auscultation • Respiratory distress with wheeze

Figure 5.5 Significant factors to consider for diagnosis

When to conduct an X-ray for children with suspected LRTI:

- If an inhaled foreign body is suspected
- If a LRTI is recurrent despite appropriate treatment
- If the X-ray will alter your management

If the child is unwell enough to require admission, then the paediatric medical team can decide whether an X-ray is indicated.

Figure 5.6 When to conduct an X-ray for children with suspected lower respiratory tract infection (LRTI)

Generally, children fall into one of the following three categories:

1. **A child who has a cough and crackles in the chest, but is not in respiratory distress and is not unwell, is unlikely to have a significant LRTI.**
2. **A child who has cough and fever and focal crepitations in the chest, but no distress, probably has a LRTI.**
3. **A child with cough, fever and respiratory distress has a LRTI until proven otherwise, particularly if there is a focal finding in the chest.**

Management

Most children with LRTIs are managed with oral antibiotics at home. Below is a list of factors which should prompt you to consider referral or to seek advice from a paediatrician:

- Age under two years old. If a child of this age has pneumonia, they are usually unwell.
- Moderate respiratory distress. These children often benefit from supplemental oxygen.
- Any signs of sepsis or dehydration ie tachycardia, pale, or significantly unwell.
- Any floppy episodes or blue episodes.
- Poor fluid intake or any vomiting, as this will make it unlikely that oral medication will be successful.
- Fevers >39°C, or fevers unresponsive to adequate doses of antipyretics.
- Oxygen saturations of <93%.
- Any underlying chronic lung disease, not including asthma. If a child has a LRTI and an exacerbation of asthma, then it is still reasonable to manage both without referral as long as each of the two aspects would have been treated outside of hospital independent of each other.
- Parental anxiety despite a full explanation.

Children who can be managed at home on oral antibiotics are usually those who have a

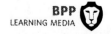

cough, fever and focal chest signs but have not yet developed respiratory distress or become particularly unwell. Although there are many factors to take into consideration, **you can usually tell who is well enough to be managed at home just by looking at them.**

Unlike with adults, a follow-up is not often needed. If a parent is advised that the cough will improve with the antibiotics and may take a couple of weeks to go altogether, then they should also be advised to seek a review if one of those two things does not happen.

How to be a know-it-all

As mentioned previously, over-reliance on chest signs can be very misleading in trying to decide who does and doesn't have a chest infection. One sign that does seem to point towards a bacterial LRTI in younger children in particular is **grunting**. Children grunt when there is an element of collapse in the lungs. The grunt is an involuntary partial closure of the glottis which keeps a small amount of pressure in the airways so that they do not collapse at the end of expiration.

It is not uncommon to see a child with what would otherwise seem to be an upper respiratory tract infection yet who grunts intermittently. The presence of grunting should prompt a careful examination to look for signs of LRTI.

What do I tell the parents?

When I do not think their child has a 'chest infection':

"Most coughs in childhood are not due to chest infections. Even when children are ruttly with a cough, it is usually due to mucous produced by a viral infection. When I examined your child I couldn't find any of the things that would indicate a chest infection. Because of this it is better if they don't have antibiotics. As you are probably aware, antibiotics can cause problems such as diarrhoea,

thrush, urine infection and allergic reactions, so we always try to make sure a child really needs them rather than just giving them 'just in case'."

"Instead, you should concentrate on giving medicines for fever if they have one. I don't think that it worth spending your money on cough medicines, because they don't work well at all."

"Most viral coughs last a few days as a severe cough and then become mild, but can stay as a nuisance cough for quite a while. However, if you think it is not getting better you should get your child seen again. Sometimes, a minor infection can come before a more significant infection, so if your child becomes worse, I would want your child to be seen again quickly."

When I think that a child has a 'chest infection' but does not need to be admitted:

"When I examined your child, some of the things that I found suggest that they have a chest infection. This is something that lots of children get at some point in their childhood and mostly they respond well to antibiotic medicine."

"I think that your child is well enough to have their medicine at home. It may take a day for any improvement to be noticeable. If they are no better then, or if they are significantly worse at any point then they need to be seen again to see if they need to have any different treatment. You should not hesitate to get your child seen again if you are worried."

When I think that a child has a 'chest infection' and I feel that they need admission:

"Your child has the signs of a chest infection. As doctors, we call this pneumonia*. Pneumonia is not as dangerous to children as it is to old people, so you shouldn't worry about it in the same way. Most children respond very well to antibiotics including children who are poorly enough to need hospital treatment."

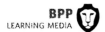

"Because your child is quite unwell with their infection, I would like them to be seen by the paediatricians. They will decide what treatment your child needs to have."

*NB. I always try to make sure that I use the word 'pneumonia' with parents early on. It carries a real fear of death and they will hear it used later on. If you don't explain it to them, no one else might. When parents are not spoken to openly, they often assume that this is because the doctors do not want to tell them that their child might die. Of course, they may have someone explain things well to them later, but they may still be upset that you only told them that their child had a chest infection when the 'specialist' diagnosed pneumonia!

Flowchart for managing lower respiratory tract infection

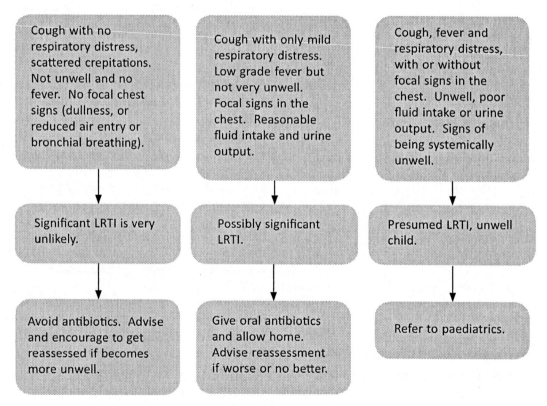

Figure 5.7 Flowchart for managing lower respiratory tract infection

Summary for lower respiratory tract infection (LRTI)

- LRTI usually manifests as cough with fever and respiratory distress. Focal chest signs make the diagnosis more likely but are not always present.
- Children with cough and bilateral crackles without fever or respiratory distress probably have a viral illness and are therefore unlikely to benefit from antibiotics. Focal crackles in a child without other features of LRTI can be due to the mucous produced by viral infections.
- Most children with LRTI can be managed at home on oral antibiotics. Those who require assessment with a view to admission can usually be identified by looking at them. They look unwell, tired or significantly distressed.

5.2 Urinary tract infection (UTI)

Assessment

Assessing and treating UTI in children is very different to the way that it is managed in adults. This is because it is more difficult to diagnose as there are rarely specific symptoms, children are more likely to have an underlying urinary tract anatomical abnormality and children are more prone to complications of UTI such as renal scarring.

In order to correctly manage this condition, getting the first step right is the most important. Obtaining appropriate specimens, testing them and interpreting them are vital to making the correct diagnosis as well as to guiding treatment and further investigations. Failure to do this adequately will mislead the physician and allow wrong diagnoses to be made. Additionally it will not ensure appropriate antibiotics are given and may lead to unnecessary testing or lack of appropriate investigations.

The most common reason for obtaining urine specimens in children is because we need to rule out a urine infection. This is in contrast to the 10–70-year-old age group where we tend to test urines to confirm a strongly suspected diagnosis of UTI. Because of this different dynamic,

misleading results in younger children cause far more trouble to doctors, parents and patients. The worst possible situation occurs when a suspected UTI is treated with no specimen obtained at all prior to starting treatment in a young child. This makes life very hard when trying to decide what to do when the patient doesn't respond to treatment and also leaves uncertainty about the need for investigations even if they do get better.

The ideal specimen in most circumstances is a clean catch specimen obtained prior to starting antibiotics. For a small child, this involves cleaning the perineum, and then sitting the child on an adult's knee with a sterile collection pot or bowl. Although it reduces the likelihood of contamination, this can be an anxious process and some children will actually withhold passing urine while their nappy is off. For the older child who can pass urine on demand, this method of collection is more straightforward.

If a clean catch is not possible then a pad method can be used, provided that the equipment is genuinely kept sterile apart from being placed in the nappy. Urine bags are an alternative but are prone to spilling and to contamination. With pads and bags, it is essential to collect the urine as soon as the child has passed urine, as prolonged contact with the skin is going to make contamination more likely.

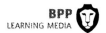

With younger children and more unwell children, there is a high likelihood that the diagnosis of UTI will mean that the child goes on to have imaging of the urinary tract. Because of this factor it is good practice with any UTI (other than a first UTI in a healthy child over three years old) to **obtain two specimens prior to starting treatment.** This will protect the child from uncertainty and enduring inappropriate investigations when just one specimen is sent and is found to be contaminated.

Even once specimens are obtained, diagnosis is rarely straightforward. Ideally, there will be a dipstick test with +++ leukocytes (white cells) and which is positive for nitrites. However in the absence of a dipstick which tests strongly positive, interpretation is complicated by the following factors:

- Minor febrile illnesses (such as URTI) in children cause red and white blood cells to 'leak' into the urinary tract. 1–2 'pluses' of leukocytes may result from this.
- **In younger children urine dipsticks are less reliable.** This is because the reagents on the stick do not always test positive if urine has not been held in the bladder for a reasonable amount of time. For this reason, children who are not toilet-trained may not test positive on dipstick testing.
- Nappy rash and an inflamed perineum from repeated wiping may cause red and white cells in the urine.
- Because of the two factors above, a nitrite positive dipstick is supposed to be more specific, however it is also difficult to interpret when nitrite testing is positive in the absence of leukocytes.
- Children can develop other reasons for having positive dipsticks, precisely at the times of non-specific febrile illness. Nephrotic syndrome can follow an URTI and causes proteinuria +/- haematuria. Henoch-Schonlein purpura causes haematuria and even causes abdominal pain!

Management

A decision has to be made based on the overall picture. It is also important to consider whether another more serious infection such as meningitis could be partially treated by prescribing antibiotics. A good degree of certainty is the aim, and then, once a provisional diagnosis is made, you can treat the UTI. Choice of the type of antibiotic should be guided by local sensitivities which can be advised upon by the microbiology lab which you use. The route of administration will be oral in most cases, however, consider referring the child for assessment by a paediatrician with a view to having intravenous antibiotics in the following situations.

Consider urgent referral if:

- Age under three months (I would say that this is a 'must do')
- Age under twelve months (if in doubt, discuss these with a paediatrician)
- Vomiting or unable to tolerate medicines orally
- Unwell, tachycardic or any signs of systemic upset
- Any history of a funny turn or floppy episode during the illness
- Poor fluid intake

Finally, a follow-up needs to be organised. The most important aspect of aftercare is to ensure that the child gets better and that the final lab result of the urine specimen is reviewed. The latter is important because it may be that despite a dipstick suggestive of UTI, no bacteria is grown, or that a bacteria is grown and is not sensitive to the first line antibiotics. Remember that **if you have done a test, you are responsible for acting upon it.** It is therefore vital to either arrange a follow-up within your own team or if, for example, you are asking the child's own

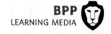

GP to follow this up, that you should speak to someone and arrange this.*

If a UTI could be treated without admission and responds to first line oral antibiotics quickly, then it is unlikely to need any further investigations or treatment. Opinions are divided on this subject and it is important to know which guidelines are being used by your local paediatric outpatients to determine investigations. Many have started using the National Institute for Health and Clinical Excellence (NICE) guidelines, however many hospitals are using their own guidelines. What is important to understand is the reason for investigations. Tests are needed to ensure that:

- There is no underlying (anatomical) abnormality which has predisposed to the development of a UTI.
- The UTI has not caused any renal impairment or scarring.

Underlying abnormalities and renal scarring are more likely if:

- The child is younger
- The child was more unwell during the UTI
- The UTI did not quickly respond to treatment
- The bacteria grown was not pure e-coli
- This was not the child's first UTI

---

*A note here for any hospital doctors reading this book. All the GPs that I know are very happy to be more involved with the care of their own patients. What they don't like is having to follow through what was started in secondary care with inadequate information and no guidance. Try not to send patients away with instructions to see their GPs for follow up/tests/treatment. Parents will forget 90% of what you say but they won't tell their GP this. So they will turn up at the GP surgery, demand to be seen and tell a tale of how no one explained anything to them at hospital. This will, of course seem quite credible as a possibility to the GP who now has to 'do something' but doesn't know what is expected of them.

In general, these factors should prompt referral or discussion for advice about local practice with regard to following up children who have had a proven UTI.

Instead, try writing a letter for the patient to take, or even better, phone the GP. Receptionists will usually move heaven and earth for you because 'a specialist' has phoned. The GP will be so amazed that they got a phone call, instead of an unhelpful computer-generated letter several months later, that they will agree to most requests. They will have the opportunity to ask questions and may even have some useful information for you about the patient.

De-mystifying the role of the paediatrician: what the paediatrician might do

- The management of straightforward UTIs in the paediatric assessment unit is essentially no different to the way that they are managed in a general practice or emergency department setting. The only two ways that paediatricians are likely to have a different approach is to do with specimens and blood pressure measurement.
- Because we paediatricians are conditioned by seeing children who were treated for UTI but either had no confirmatory or no uncontaminated specimen obtained, we are often more rigorous about obtaining specimens. This, coupled with the fact that we are more comfortable doing procedures such as catheterisation and supra-pubic aspiration, means that we tend to spend more effort to ensure obtaining an adequate urine specimen.
- Secondly, because we have the equipment and staff to achieve this, we usually check blood pressures in children who present with UTI. This additional information is useful in raising suspicion that a child may have

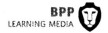

had repeated and undiagnosed UTIs previously. This scenario is one which is still seen too often and commonly results in scarring of the kidneys.

How to be a know-it-all

The easiest thing to forget when dealing with a child who has had a UTI is (to remember) to consider whether there is an avoidable underlying factor contributing to the child prone developing UTIs. One factor which can predispose a child to UTI is poor fluid intake, especially during hot weather, although the condition which so commonly goes hand in hand with UTI is constipation.

The way that this works is that any prolonged carriage of faeces in the rectum can affect bladder voiding. If the bladder does not empty fully when the child voids then bacteria have a better chance of culturing in the urinary bladder. It is therefore important to always ask about symptoms of constipation (see Chapter 9) and also to have a lower threshold for diagnosing and treating constipation. After all, in a child who has had a UTI, constipation cannot be considered to be either sub-clinical or worth watching to see if it goes away on its own.

FAQs

What do I do with this result? The urine has grown e-coli/a mixed growth, but the test was done two weeks ago and the child is better now. No antibiotics were given.

This is a common scenario, which is best avoided by ensuring that all urine cultures are reviewed two days after they are sent to the lab. Even then, a positive result can be found after a child has become asymptomatic.

The first thing to do is to consider the credibility of the result. Is it a pure growth of single bacteria? Was there significant pyuria? Next, contact the

parent and find out how the child is. Are they completely back to their normal selves? Even if this is the case, the child may well have had a UTI and fought it off, or the infection may now be sub-clinical.

If the child is completely well, you should obtain a repeat specimen and await the result. If the first specimen was contaminated, it is doubly important to make sure that a good clean specimen is collected this time and goes quickly to the labs. Do not start treatment if the child is well because if this repeat specimen is ambiguous, antibiotics will further complicate the matter.

If the child sounds as though they may well have a UTI, the repeat specimen should be dipstick tested and, if suggestive of UTI, treated as above. If in doubt, discuss with a paediatrician. After all, they may be seeing this child as an outpatient eventually.

What do I tell the parents?

When I have diagnosed UTI in a child who is well and can be treated at home:

"The urine specimen which we have tested has shown signs that there is probably a urine infection. This is a lot like 'cystitis' in an adult. In children it can be difficult to tell that they have a urine infection, which is why it was so important to get this specimen for us to test. The test that we have done gives us some indications of a urine infection. I will also be sending it to the lab for confirmation that there is an infection."

"Because your child is not too unwell, I am going to prescribe them an antibiotic which they can take at home. We have to use an antibiotic which works against most bacteria, and this will have a noticeable effect in the next twenty-four hours if it is going to work. If it isn't working, then the urine specimen which I am sending to the labs will tell us which antibiotic to use next. Because we are relying on these results, I find that it is safer to get a second urine specimen before starting the antibiotics.

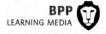

However, if your child can't do one straight away, we could give you the pot and let you get the second specimen at home. This then needs to come back to us straightaway or if not, stay in the fridge until you can bring it to us."

"Most children who get urine infections get them for no reason. You do not need to worry that you could have done anything to stop this from happening. Usually, this will be a one-off infection, though some children will have more. Now that you have had this experience, it will help you make sure that your child has a urine specimen tested the next time that they are unwell."

"Deciding what tests or further treatment is needed will depend on the results of the urine specimens, so you need to... [Follow-up can be arranged as appropriate, but should generally be with someone who has access to the details of the illness, and the urine result and should take place when the antibiotics are finished. Follow-up can be over the phone.] *As I mentioned before, I am expecting these antibiotics to work, however if you feel that they are not helping you should contact...* [access to a phone number where advice can be sought is vital in case the child is worse or no better.]"

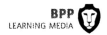

Flowchart for assessing the child with a urinary tract infection

Suspect UTI in most unwell children, unless a clear focus for infection is found elsewhere. Even if another focus is found, UTI may still be present.

Obtain a urine specimen. Start this process early, as it may take some time. For small children, aim to get a 'clean catch' urine from a clean, naked child.

Urine dipstick testing.

Unclear or borderline result.

Consider other explanations (eg nappy rash) and obtain a second specimen, which may be clearer. If UTI is the most likely diagnosis, treat as such when two good specimens are obtained. Uncertainty will be answered by the urine culture result.

Positive result.

Refer to local or national guidelines for treatment. Referral or at least paediatric involvement is likely to be needed if: age under twelve months old; vomiting or unable to tolerate medicines orally; unwell, tachycardic or any signs of systemic upset; any history of a funny turn or floppy episode during the illness; poor fluid intake.

If the child can be treated as an outpatient, take responsibility for making sure the urine culture result is reviewed as soon as it is available. Review the child one way or another at the time that the antibiotics finish or sooner if the child is worse/no better. Consider obtaining a repeat urine culture 48 hours after antibiotics have finished to ensure adequate treatment. Refer to local or national guidelines regarding need for investigations.

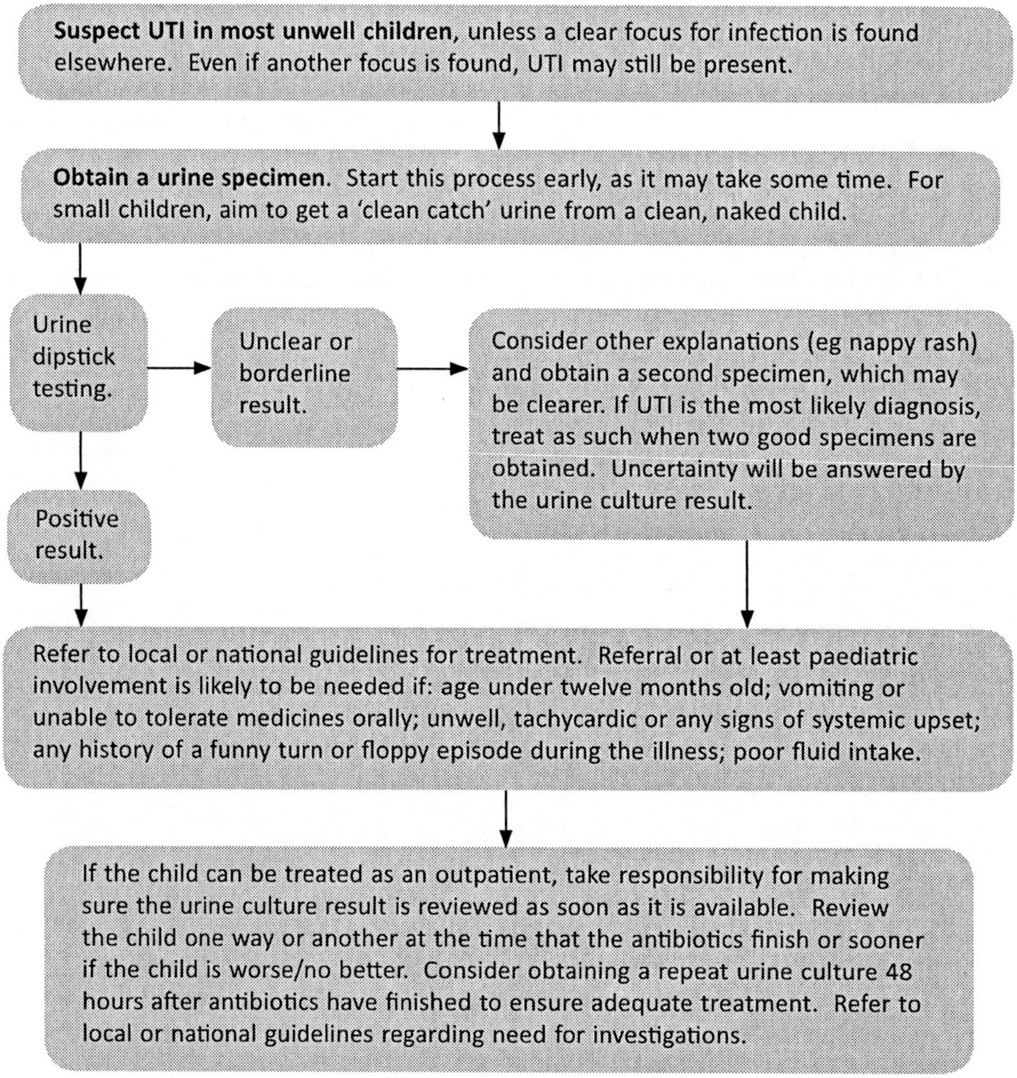

Figure 5.8 Flowchart for assessing the child with a urinary tract infection

Summary for urinary tract infection (UTI)

- UTI is treated differently in children and the younger the child, the more significant an event it is.
- The most important step in managing UTI is to rule it out in any child who is unwell and does not have a clear focus for infection (such as an otitis media).
- In order to diagnose UTI, at least one good urine specimen should be dipsticked, and if positive, sent for culture.
- Most UTIs respond to first line oral antibiotics. Local or national guidelines (eg NICE guidelines) should be used to decide about treatment and investigations.

5.3 Meningitis

Assessment

- Although thankfully becoming rarer in the UK since the introduction of the MenC vaccine, **meningitis is still one of the most feared children's illnesses.**
- For the purposes of the initial assessment, **meningitis is a clinical diagnosis** which may or may not be confirmed later on lumbar puncture.
- In some cases cerebrospinal fluid is never obtained and so **the clarity and documentation of the initial assessment will have significant impact on the future care of that child**. This is especially true for the doctor giving the first dose of antibiotics.

The way that meningitis manifests depends on the age of the child; in each case, however, the same process is at work. The inflammation of the lining of the brain (meninges) causes the child to be unsettled and irritable. The fever and the toxins produced by the infection affect the child's level of consciousness. Finally there may or may not be systemic upset manifested as tachycardia and poor perfusion of the hands and feet. This will depend on whether the child has purely meningitis or meningitis with sepsis. When a child has both, either one can manifest before the other.

Suspect meningitis when:

- There is **poor feeding** (babies) or poor fluid intake (in older children). Minor illnesses will almost always put children off their food but generally they will continue to drink just enough. If a child stops drinking all together, they are probably very unwell and meningitis should be strongly suspected.
- **A child will not settle.** Irritability is different from being miserable. A miserable child tends to settle with a cuddle and responds to simple analgesia, while an irritable child wants to be left alone and becomes more

unhappy when handled. A miserable child is purposeful in their misery (pushes you away or hides their face) while an irritable child is random in their unhappiness.
- There are signs of **meningial irritation**. This includes back arching in babies, increased tone at all ages, neck stiffness in older children, and photophobia (although this is more commonly seen in the teenage group).
- **Reduced level of consciousness (see introductory chapter).**
- There has been **recent contact** with a child who has or is suspected to have meningococcal infection.
- Signs of **sepsis**.

When your assessment is complete you will have an index of suspicion about the possibility that the child has bacterial meningitis. As the assessing doctor, it is helpful to separate these children into three groups:

1. Likely.
2. Possible.
3. Not suspected.

Children who likely have meningitis rarely present. When they do, they are quite unwell and the signs are usually present when they are looked for. The younger child will be inconsolable and have increased tone. The older child may have classic neck stiffness and photophobia.

To avoid missing the occasional case of meningitis that most doctors will see from time to time, you have to consider far more children to potentially have meningitis than actually do. The children who fall into this category have no clear evidence of meningitis but 'are not their normal selves'. They are not unwell enough to prompt urgent action but they don't seem well enough to dismiss and discharge back to the parents' care immediately. This group is a difficult group because of course children are not their normal selves when they are poorly,

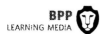

so the vast majority of children who are having an 'off day' have a minor illness rather than a serious infection such as meningitis. The key to sorting these children out from the dozens afflicted by simple viral URTI is to look for the signs above, and if possible see how the child progresses or, even better, how they respond to medication.

For children who seem most likely to have a straightforward viral infection, but could possibly have a serious infection such as meningitis, the safest strategy is to delay your decision for about an hour. During this time, you should ensure that the child has had the maximum amount of antipyretic medication allowed and is offered fluids frequently. Most children will be reassuringly on the upward, improving slope of the usual fluctuation seen in minor illnesses, allowing you to put meningitis into the unlikely category.

The vast majority of children do not have meningitis and, after careful assessment, you will be able to mentally classify them as 'unlikely' to have meningitis. I use this word because **most children who present with meningitis have had a prodromal upper respiratory tract infection**. This means that should the parents have seen a doctor and expressed concerns regarding meningitis, it will be very awkward if that doctor declared that the child did not have meningitis, even though that doctor was right at that moment in time. It is good practice to consider any minor illness as a prodrome to more severe infection, and ensure good 'safety-netting' when advising parents.

Management

Many children with meningitis will have sepsis simultaneously. The management of sepsis is outlined later in this chapter, while this section deals with meningitis without sepsis.

For children who likely have meningitis, the two most important things for an assessing doctor

to do are to **ensure that the child receives antibiotics as soon as possible and that they are seen by an experienced paediatrician quickly**. The order in which these two things occur depend on your working environment. If you work in close proximity to the paediatric team, then it is probably better to make an urgent referral and allow them to decide whether antibiotics will be given before or after a lumbar puncture is performed. Your job is to refer to someone who makes it clear that they have understood that you feel this child *has* meningitis, rather than *may have*. The person who takes the referral should now make your patient an immediate priority.

If, however, you are in a position where you strongly suspect meningitis but the child will face a significant wait before seeing the paediatricians then antibiotic administration should not be delayed. You should still refer the child but also give a formulary dose of intramuscular (IM) or intravenous (IV) broad spectrum antibiotics. Most commonly, this is in the form of intramuscular benzyl penicillin in general practice and intravenous cefalosporins in the emergency department. The decision to do this can be discussed with the paediatricians. However, only you have actually seen the child, so I would be cautious about being discouraged from giving antibiotics by a doctor on the other end of the phone who is not responsible for the outcome of your decision. Allow yourself to be persuaded if the advice seems appropriate, but ultimately you need to take the responsibility for giving or not giving antibiotics prior to transferring the child.

What do I tell the parents?

When I feel that a child is well enough to go home, but I want the parents to be wary for signs of meningitis:

"Having examined/observed your child, I am satisfied that they have an infection that is not dangerous and does not need hospital treatment. I do not expect them to be completely well.

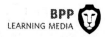

Most children who have minor infections go through periods of being a bit worse and then a bit better. They also usually respond well to medicines for fever such as paracetamol. The children that I usually worry about are the children who get a bit worse and then get worse again or don't get any better."

"There are some things that you should look out for, such as being floppy, unable to drink, or developing a rash that doesn't go pale when you stretch the skin. These things would tell you that you need to get your child seen by a doctor again. However, I think that the most important reason why a child should be seen again is because a parent feels that something new is wrong, even if you can't put your finger on what it is. If you are worried, you should [advise the parents according to the local set up]. Do not hesitate to seek advice again. No one will think that you are being too anxious."

When I think that a child needs referral for possible meningitis:

"I can see that you are quite worried about how ill your child is. When I examined them they appear quite poorly to me as well. It is difficult to be sure whether they really do have a serious infection and what that serious infection is. Because children who are this poorly can have infections such as meningitis, we err on the side of caution and treat with antibiotics. We need to do this because it is harmful to wait if a child does have a serious infection, although it does mean that sometimes we are treating a child who just has a very bad flu bug."

"So now I am going to refer to the hospital doctors / give some antibiotics to your child. Then the hospital doctors can assess more fully and make sure that all the necessary tests are done to be sure what the infection is."

"You don't need to worry that this has happened because of anything that you have done or haven't done. You have brought your child to us when they became poorly, which was the right thing to do. If you had brought them earlier, we probably would have only found a cold and sent you away again."

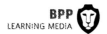

Flowchart for assessing the child with meningitis

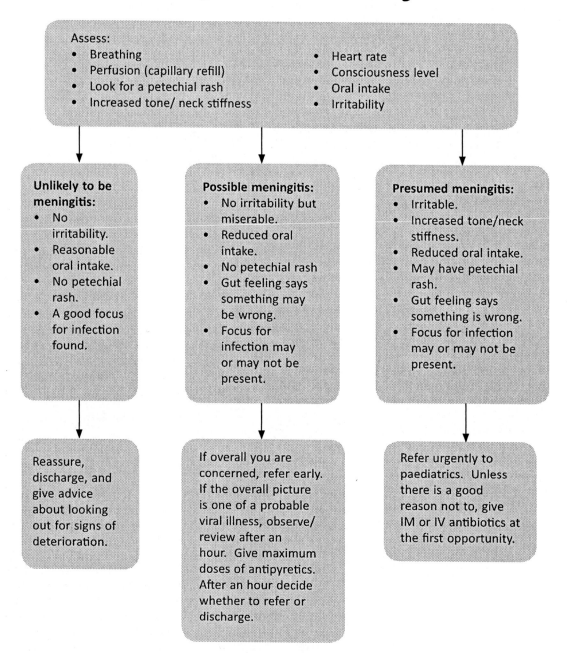

Figure 5.9 Flowchart for assessing the child with meningitis

Summary for meningitis

- Meningitis is a condition which rarely occurs in children.
- Meningitis can cause disability or death.
- Early recognition and treatment improve outcome.
- Symptoms of meningitis are often vague and may be blamed on other illnesses.
- In babies, signs of meningitis may be as non-specific as poor feeding.
- Meningitis should always be suspected in the moderately unwell child.
- Some signs such as irritable cry, back arching, refusal to feed, increased tone, and neck stiffness or photophobia are highly suspicious of meningitis in a febrile child.
- Unless meningitis is excluded as a possibility, the safest strategy is to observe and review a child or refer for further assessment.
- Children with apparent meningitis should be given intramuscular penicillin or intravenous cephalosporin as soon as the diagnosis is made, unless they are going to be seen by the paediatric team within minutes.

5.4 Sepsis

Assessment

- Sepsis is the physiological state caused by systemic infection, which is usually bacterial in this context.
- Sepsis usually has a 'parent' infection which can be serious in its own right such as meningitis.
- Other causes include urinary tract infection (UTI), abscesses and pneumonia. However, because the bacteria that cause sepsis can be found in the nasopharynx as commensals, invasive infection can occur without an apparent focus being present.
- It is unclear why bacteria will survive in a sub-clinical state in the majority of cases and then occasionally cause severe life-threatening infections.

The child who is developing or has developed sepsis may therefore have the signs and symptoms of a focal infection such as a UTI. The signs of sepsis itself are to do with the systemic upset caused by the way that the infection affects the child's physiology. Essentially, toxins produced by the bacteria cause the blood vessels to lose tone. This causes poor perfusion of tissues and leaking of fluid from the vascular system into the tissues, which further worsens delivery of oxygen and nutrients. Each organ has a different way of showing that it is no longer well perfused and the signs of inadequate perfusion should be sought in any unwell child.

Because the body prioritises vital organ perfusion, **the first effects of septic shock are seen in the skin.** When the beginnings of sepsis manifest, the child will become pale, their heart rate will increase and capillary refill time will be prolonged. Note that babies and cold children (as most children are in the UK if they have been taken to see the doctor on most days of the year) will have delayed capillary refill in the hands and feet. This will improve when the child is warm again. Capillary refill is best tested by pressing firmly on the sternum for five seconds, releasing, and then counting how many seconds it takes for colour to completely return to that of the surrounding tissues. Anything over two seconds is considered significant as long as it is taken in context of the child and the other findings from the examination.

Next, the body will start to try to maintain perfusion to the heart and brain by reducing flow to the abdominal organs. For this reason,

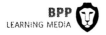

poor urine output is one sign of severe sepsis. Although urine output is sometimes difficult to assess in this context, it is important to ask about urine output that day.

The child's physiology is designed to maintain blood flow to the heart and brain at all cost. It is therefore important to realise that **when a child with sepsis is drowsy, subdued or agitated, the sepsis is life-threatening.** By this point, the child will be very tachycardic, most likely pale and have poor tone.

Another aspect of identifying sepsis is the hunt for the petechial rash. When present, petechiae or purpuric spots can indicate meningococcal infection. It is therefore important to look for any marks that do not blanch when pressed. It is equally important of course not to be caught out by mistaking moles, or artefacts such as marker pen drawings, for petechiae!

Management

Once recognised, **the septic child needs antibiotics and fluid resuscitation as soon as possible.** Children are very good at compensating for any deficit in circulating volume but these compensatory mechanisms are crippled by the toxins that produce sepsis. When a child is showing the signs of cardiovascular compromise, they have already got approximately a 25% deficit in their circulation.

By this point oral resuscitation will no longer suffice. The child needs intravenous fluids and antibiotics. The management of the child will therefore depend on the setting which the child is in.

In a general practice setting, a child with signs of sepsis should be transferred by emergency ambulance to the nearest emergency department. If any petechiae are present, the child should be given intramuscular benzyl penicillin as soon as this can be made up, and this dosage should be communicated to the receiving hospital.

In the emergency department, the child should be cannulated and blood taken for full blood count, Urea and electrolytes, C-reactive protein and a blood culture. If possible, a clotting screen will help the paediatricians as well. The child with any signs of shock should receive a 20ml/kg fluid bolus of an isotonic fluid such as normal saline. At the same time, a senior paediatric doctor should be informed and a member of the paediatric team should come to assist with the child's care urgently.

The 'must do's

☑ Always check a blood sugar. (Remember that glucagon is no good to a hypoglycaemic child. They have no glycogen left to release.)

☑ Always look for signs of sepsis in a child who is not their normal cheerful self.

☑ **Aim to give fluids and antibiotics early;** usually, this means giving them yourself

Pitfalls to avoid

☒ Never take a risk and send a child home unless you are satisfied with them systemically.

☒ Never hesitate to ask for help and advice with managing poorly children.

☒ Beware the child on oral antibiotics, especially if the history suggests that they were prescribed without a clear indication. Such children may have a partially treated sepsis.

How to be a know-it-all

There are many causes of non-blanching spots and rashes and the majority of children with petechiae do not have meningococcal sepsis. However, because meningococcal infection is such an important diagnosis to exclude, doctors quite rightly worry when they find petechial lesions. When a child has petechiae or purpura

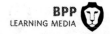

and is unwell and febrile, it is straightforward that they should be treated for presumed meningococcal infection. Even then, not all of these children will be proven to have had the infection. The key to identifying the child who does not need treating for possible sepsis is to understand the other causes for non-blanching lesions, and also to appreciate the reason for the petechial rash in sepsis. The rash exists for two reasons. Firstly, the rash is an inflammatory phenomenon, causing a vasculitis. Secondly, the rash can be due to subcutaneous capillary leakage due to deranged clotting. Both of these causes of the petechiae and purpura seen in sepsis are due to toxins produced by the bacteria. It would therefore be difficult to explain how a child is healthy and yet manifests a petechial rash due to meningococcal infection. Although malignancy and clotting disorders are worth thinking about as possibilities, they are very unlikely in the context of an acute presentation if there are no suggestive features in the history (such as weight loss or a previous history of significant bleeding). The other possibilities and how to recognise them are listed below.

Artefactual. Minor grazes, pen marks and chocolate have all been mistaken for petechiae on repeated occasions. As well as testing to see if a mark blanches, it is well worth trying to wipe off a lesion to see if it comes away. A true petechial spot is purple in colour and can be distinguished from these pretenders when they are closely examined.

Mechanical. Increased venous pressure will caused capillaries to burst and can produce the most spectacular petechial rashes. The children with mechanical petechiae will be identifiable from two features which will usually be quite striking. Firstly, the rash will consist of lots of tiny spots. There are never purpura in these cases. The rash is usually impressively confluent, although the petechiae may be sparse and still be due to a mechanical cause. Secondly, the rash will be localised depending on the mechanism. The most common patterns seen are:

- Head, neck, arms and chest above the nipples. This is due to coughing, vomiting or straining which has raised the pressure in the superior vena cava.
- Distal part of a limb due to rough play, abuse, or a tourniquet.
- The head only. This distribution is suggestive of throttling if dramatic but limited to the head. Occasional petechiae on the face can still be due to coughing or vomiting.
- The lower limbs of a baby. I have seen this occur with nappies that are applied too tightly.
- An isolated patch anywhere on the body due to a blunt injury. This can be due to any localised trauma.
- Circular patches on the limbs of a child. This may be due to sucking the skin, a peculiar childhood pastime. If this is the case, all the lesions will be in clusters the size of an open mouth and occur on skin that the child can place in their mouth.

When a pattern is recognised, an explanation that would match the pattern can be sought. If this is the case, no tests or treatment are needed. Remember that this may be the presentation of a non-accidental injury.

Immune Thrombocytopaenia Purpura (ITP). This condition is an autoimmune disease which usually follows a trivial viral infection. Antibodies produced in response to the infection destroy platelets at an impressive rate, leading to the development of petechiae and occasionally purpura. The child is usually quite well and may even no longer have the original viral infection. Fortunately the child's ability to produce new platelets remains intact, so these children rarely come to any harm. The diagnosis is usually obvious by the fact that a child is well and yet has an impressive number of petechiae. Confirmation is made by doing a full blood count, which will show a platelet count below 50 in most cases. The full blood count is also a useful test in these cases to pick up the very rare cases of leukaemia. I think that abnormal blood

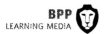

counts are best discussed with a paediatrician, whether they are referred or not.

Henoch-Schönlein Purpura (HSP). This disease usually causes a purpuric rash on the buttocks and the extensor surfaces of the lower limbs. When there is purpura in this distribution, the diagnosis is usually obvious. However, the rash can begin as a petechial rash and may be found elsewhere, so this is an important diagnosis to consider in the child who has petechiae and no fever. When this condition is suspected, involve the paediatricians, since HSP can involve the kidneys.

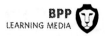

What do I tell the parents?

The assessment of your child suggests that they may be fighting a serious infection. Sometimes the signs of the more significant infections are very vague. If an infection is taking hold then it is important to start antibiotics straight away even if we cannot be sure yet.

The tests which will tell us for sure about infection take two or three days to be complete, so you should expect to be in hospital for at least this long. On the whole, children respond very quickly to antibiotics, or turn out to have had severe viral infections which get better on their own. Because it is impossible to be sure at this stage which children are going to have the most dangerous infections, the safest thing to do is to start antibiotics through a drip, do all the necessary tests and watch them very carefully over the next day or so

Flowchart for assessing the child with possible sepsis

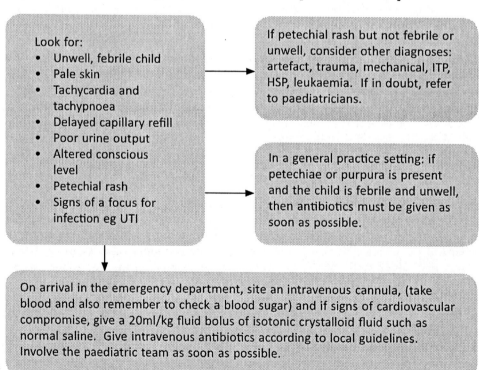

Look for:
- Unwell, febrile child
- Pale skin
- Tachycardia and tachypnoea
- Delayed capillary refill
- Poor urine output
- Altered conscious level
- Petechial rash
- Signs of a focus for infection eg UTI

If petechial rash but not febrile or unwell, consider other diagnoses: artefact, trauma, mechanical, ITP, HSP, leukaemia. If in doubt, refer to paediatricians.

In a general practice setting: if petechiae or purpura is present and the child is febrile and unwell, then antibiotics must be given as soon as possible.

On arrival in the emergency department, site an intravenous cannula, (take blood and also remember to check a blood sugar) and if signs of cardiovascular compromise, give a 20ml/kg fluid bolus of isotonic crystalloid fluid such as normal saline. Give intravenous antibiotics according to local guidelines. Involve the paediatric team as soon as possible.

Figure 5.10 Flowchart for assessing the child with possible sepsis

Summary for sepsis

- Sepsis is a systemic physiological insult that is usually caused by bacterial infection.
- Sepsis can occur with or without a focal infection being also present.
- Sepsis can be recognised by looking for:
  - Pale skin
  - Tachycardia and tachypnoea
  - Delayed capillary refill
  - Poor urine output
  - Altered conscious level
  - Petechial rash
- While the signs that can be seen in the skin occur early, altered conscious level indicates an advanced stage of cardiovascular shut-down.
- The most important aspect of managing sepsis is to recognise it and ensure early treatment with intravenous fluids and antibiotics.

De-mystifying the role of the paediatrician: what the paediatrician might do

- Because almost all febrile children present directly to primary care or the emergency department, the majority are also managed in this setting. It would be impossible for a paediatric service to cope if all febrile children were referred for assessment; however, paediatricians are a valuable resource when dealing with an unwell febrile child.
- As children can be difficult to assess it is often valuable to reassess them after antipyretics or a brief period of observation. The second opinion of an experienced colleague is a far better tactic than lab tests in most cases. This could be another GP, emergency medic or a paediatrician. Referral for uncertainty is better than having a child come back in extremis.
- Babies in particular can be deceptive. Many can be assessed and discharged without referral but some babies will concern the assessing doctor. Every winter it becomes the job of the paediatric medical team to reassess these babies. Current practice in paediatrics is to 'err on the side of caution' and do a full septic screen before starting broad spectrum antibiotics. Many of these babies will be discharged home three days later if all tests prove negative.

 FAQs

If I give a dose of paracetamol or ibuprofen, will I mask a serious infection?

It is not the treatment of symptoms that prevents clinicians from detecting a serious illness. Response to paracetamol or ibuprofen can be a very useful discriminatory test. I feel that children are sometimes unfairly denied antipyretics and analgesia because there is an underlying concern that this might somehow make it difficult to spot that the child is unwell. However this assessment is best based on all the other factors outlined within this book.

Children with quite straightforward illnesses can seem disproportionately miserable. A child with a fever who cries continuously and has signs of an upper respiratory tract infection probably has earache and a sore throat.

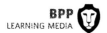

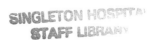

If you give them paracetamol and they start playing then I feel that this is extremely reassuring.

The danger of giving medication comes mainly if there is no focus found and the child is discharged without appropriate investigation, observation or safety-netting. I would advise that you should always obtain a urine sample as a UTI does not always cause systemic symptoms other than fever to begin with.

The other group of patients who should never be treated blindly with antipyretics is small babies. It is unusual for babies under the age of a few months to get infections at all and the proportion that proves to be serious is greater in this age group.

If there is good evidence for a viral illness then that can be treated with simple antipyretics alone. However, it is uncommon for babies to require such medications so it is always best to be sure of what you are treating.

The answer is that **if the child has been properly assessed it is inappropriate to withhold medication and quite likely to help your assessment** (or the assessment of the paediatrician who can come and say 'this child looks really well'). If a child is brought to us by parents who have given paracetamol at home and the child looks completely well, we do not do a full septic screen and start antibiotics in case there is a masked infection, so why should we withhold medication if it has not yet been given?

Chapter 6
Abdominal pain

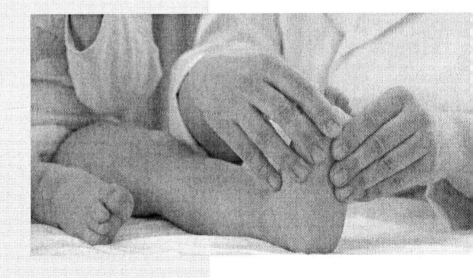

Abdominal pain

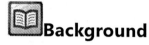

Background

Abdominal pain is a frequent occurrence in children of all ages. There are endless possible causes for abdominal pain, most of which are harmless. Often, the pathology is not even in the abdomen. Younger children in particular have a tendency to complain of abdominal pain when completely unrelated parts of their body are suffering the true insult. Middle ear infections are one such common reason for a toddler to say that their tummy hurts. In many cases the cause is never found and the pain disappears as mysteriously as it came.

Assessing the child with abdominal pain can be a very rewarding experience. Most of the time, the child will be brought to you by puzzled, anxious parents. Usually, you will be able to offer an explanation, reassurance and possibly even a treatment. So consider these children a challenge which you expect to conquer.

How to assess

Much of this is the same as assessing adults with the same problem. You take a history and then examine the child and possibly do some tests. At the end of this process you will have an idea as to whether or not there is a surgical problem and whether you know what the cause of the abdominal pain is. If you have no definite diagnosis, do not be surprised. The decision is now whether to send the child home or refer them (and to whom you will refer them).

Since you will probably want to test a urine specimen, it is worthwhile making this a priority from the start. Otherwise, when you do ask, the child will just have passed urine and then seems to lose all ability to do so for the next few hours.

Then, starting with the history, it is important to ask the following questions:

- When did the pain first appear? Has it been constant since then or does it come and go?
- Does anything make the pain better? If analgesia has been given, find out exactly what, how often and how much.
- Does anything make it worse?
- What is the pain like? Where is the pain felt? Has the pain moved?
- How bad is the pain? Some children will use words to describe the severity, and some can give it a score out of ten. A smiley/sad face chart is a useful tool for assessing severity.
- Has the child been eating and drinking? When was the last time they had anything? If you suspect a surgical problem, advise that the child should not have anything else to eat or drink for the time being.
- Has the child been opening their bowels? If not then have they passed wind? This question gets some great responses!
- Has there been any diarrhoea, blood or mucous in the stools?
- Has the child been passing urine? Is it less or more often than usual? Are there symptoms such as dysuria or eneuresis?
- Has anyone in the family had a similar problem either recently or in their own childhood?

When examining the child, be aware that the best information comes from standing back and looking at the child, preferably without them being aware that you are doing so. It is therefore very useful to casually pay attention to any observations that you can make while taking the history.

- Look at the whole child. How are they behaving? Are they subdued and still, or have you seen them move comfortably?

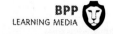

- Does the abdomen move with breathing? The younger the child, the more their abdomen will normally move while they breathe. When peritoneal discomfort sets in, this abdominal movement ceases.
- Assess skin colour, warmth of peripheries, pulse and central capillary refill.
- Listen to the chest and heart and look for signs of respiratory distress. Have you noticed a cough?
- Look at the skin of the abdomen for scars and bruises.
- Tell the child that you are about to feel their tummy. Tell them that you will be gentle and that you will stop if they want you to. Do not use the word 'hurt', even to say 'I won't hurt you.'
- While looking at the child's response, gently feel the child's abdominal wall. If the child is anxious then use their hand under yours. You will be able to assess tenderness, though not masses.
- If possible, now palpate deeply in the way that would find masses or organomegaly.
- Percuss gently, more to assess whether there is tenderness on percussion (which is a sign of peritonism) than to assess the percussion note.
- Auscultate for bowel sounds.
- Inspect the inguinal regions for hernias and in boys, inspect and palpate the scrotum.
- Now go back and examine the ears and throat. It is important to do this, since many of these children will have an upper respiratory tract infection (URTI) as the cause of their abdominal pain. To do it before examining the abdomen risks upsetting the child and will make the abdominal assessment impossible.
- Test a urine specimen and if in doubt check a blood sugar. Other tests may be helpful, but these are two tests that are relatively harmless and if not done will occasionally lead to missed diagnoses.

 # The 'must do's

- ☑ If dealing with a newborn, consider an atresia as a possibility. Even if a baby has passed meconium, there may be a congenital defect in their bowel.
- ☑ Always examine the throat and ears.
- ☑ Always check a urine specimen.
- ☑ Always examine the genitalia of a male patient.
- ☑ Always consider gynaecological causes in a pubertal female patient.
- ☑ Remember to consider child abuse at any age.
- ☑ If referring to a surgeon, remember to advise that the child should not eat or drink until they have been seen and told that they can drink again.

 # Pitfalls to avoid

- ☒ There is essentially **no role for rectal examination in children**. It should really only ever be performed in exceptional circumstances. It is not needed to assess peritonism, as that can be assessed adequately per abdomen.
- ☒ Do not avoid asking questions for fear of embarrassing the patient or parents. Better to embarrass them than suffer humiliation yourself. Do not shy away from issues of sexual activity, sexual maturity and possible abuse.
- ☒ **Do not hesitate to give adequate analgesia.** Giving a reasonable amount of painkiller will not mask significant intra-abdominal pathology and it is cruel to leave a child with untreated pain. The quantities of syrup required to give a child analgesia will not jeopardise their induction of anaesthesia should this be needed later.

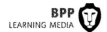

A guide to the initial management of neonatal jaundice

The information gathered will allow you to make a diagnosis in most cases. The following table lists the most common and most important diagnoses:

Diagnosis	Age group, common symptoms, etc.
Colic	This condition affects babies from soon after birth to the age of several months old. It is very common, to the extent that you could call it a normal variant. The colicky child is essentially the one who is experiencing more extreme abdominal spasms as their bowel gets used to moving food from the stomach to the rectum. It is essential to demonstrate normal growth as they present as thriving children, though the parents' may be at their wit's end. Typically they describe episodes of crying associated with drawing up of legs. This can go on for hours at a time and often nothing will settle the child. Colic can be diagnosed based on a typical history and a well child. No tests are needed, provided the child has no concerning features in the history, on examination or on the growth chart, and no treatment is effective. The management consists of reassurance and explanation.
Pyloric stenosis	This classically affects babies around the age of four weeks old. It is more common in first born males and especially where there is a family history of pyloric stenosis. **The classic history is of a progressively more severe vomiting.** The child is hungry for feeds, vomits minutes after a feed and then cries. True projectile vomiting should raise suspicion of pyloric stenosis. However, children with pyloric stenosis may not have projectile vomiting and vice versa. Surgical management is needed for this condition but usually *after* fluid resuscitation.
Intussusception	This dangerous condition can occur at any age. One peak of incidence occurs around six to twelve months of age. This is thought to be due to the child having more severe viral infections as maternal antibodies dwindle. As a result, the Peyer's patches in the gut swell in response to infection providing a lead point for the bowel to get stuck inside itself. **These children present with episodes of severe abdominal pain, or floppy and pale episodes, or both.** Vomiting is often associated. The 'textbook' sign of redcurrant jelly occurs when bowel is ischaemic and thus is a late sign. All children with suspected intussusception need urgent surgical assessment.
Constipation	The build up of faeces usually results in the symptoms of colic in children under one year old. However constipation can occur at any age and has many forms of presentation. **Constipation is a very common cause of abdominal pain in children at all ages and is frequently missed.** Because diagnosis and management of constipation is such an art form, this deserves a chapter of its very own. (See Chapter 7).
Urinary tract infection (UTI)	UTI actually rarely presents with abdominal pain in children, but it is an important differential whenever the problem is apparently abdominal. Assessment and management of UTI is covered in Chapter 5.

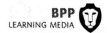

Diagnosis	Age group, common symptoms, etc.
Mesenteric Adenitis	This phenomenon occurs mainly in children under five years old. It Is abdominal pain caused by intra-abdominal lymph node inflammation and can only truly be diagnosed at laparoscopy. In reality, it is sometimes diagnosed in a child who has an obvious viral infection and associated abdominal pain. Such children are usually given analgesia and managed at home. Mesenteric adenitis can be severe however and mimic a surgical abdomen. In patients where this diagnosis is suspected but the child is more unwell, or has signs of a possible surgical abdomen, surgical assessment is compulsory even if there is a rampant upper respiratory tract infection.
Gastroenteritis	Whenever a child develops diarrhoea and vomiting due to gastroenteritis, abdominal pain can be a prominent feature. There can be colicky pains due to bowel spasms as the gut becomes inflamed. However it is the pain that follows vomiting which can lead doctors to suspect a surgical abdomen because the abdominal wall may be tender to palpation. The factors that should lead away from a diagnosis of eg appendicitis are the presence of diarrhoea, and the onset of vomiting before the pain started. Although not all abdominal tenderness is surgical, getting enough information to be sure can be difficult in children. If in doubt, observe or refer. The management of diarrhoea and vomiting is covered in Chapter 8.
Appendicitis	Appendicitis, probably the most hunted for diagnosis in the child with abdominal pain, is thankfully uncommon. It does start to occur more often in the older child and when missed can cause devastating infection. The child with mild or early appendicitis may not be easy to spot, so, when unsure, a careful assessment and repeated examination (after about an hour) are both essential. **Classic appendicitis results in an unwell and usually very subdued child.** The feature that distinguishes appendicitis from some of the causes of abdominal pain that might mimic it is the presence of abdominal pain that precedes vomiting. It is unusual to have acute appendicitis without a fever. In the older child the progression of pain from around the umbilicus towards the right lower quadrant may help to make the diagnosis. However, a textbook history is rare, and so the reality is that surgical opinions should be sought whenever a child has abdominal tenderness or other signs of a surgical abdomen.
Pneumonia	A lower lobe pneumonia is one of the causes of abdominal pain. The pneumonia is often missed initially, partly because pneumonia is sometimes difficult to pick up and partly because the chest is away from the area of focal symptoms in these patients. To avoid getting caught out, think of it as a possibility and do justice to examining the respiratory system. The management of lower respiratory tract infection is covered in Chapter 5.
Testicular torsion	About a quarter of boys who have torsion of the testes present with abdominal pain. It may also present in preverbal children who will simply be upset and inconsolable. The diagnosis is usually apparent when the scrotum is examined. The scrotum may be swollen or the testis may be tender. The important factor is to always examine the genitalia of a boy presenting with upset or abdominal pain. **Prompt surgical intervention increases the chance that the testis will be salvageable.** If the boy has the torsion corrected within four hours of onset, usually the testis will be

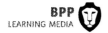

Diagnosis	Age group, common symptoms, etc.
Testicular torsion	viable. However, by twelve hours from the onset, this number has dropped below half being salvageable.
Pregnancy, ovarian torsion and pelvic inflammatory disease	I find that GPs and emergency medicine doctors are usually better than paediatricians at considering gynaecological causes for abdominal pain. About 30% of children in the UK have their first act of sexual intercourse before the age of 16. Every year approximately one in every hundred girls under the age of 16 becomes pregnant. Of course, gynaecological problems such as torsion of an ovary can occur even if not sexually active. The important thing is to realise that this is an important possibility to consider in pubertal girls. The only way to adequately assess the possibility of a gynaecological cause is to politely ask to **speak to the child alone** or with a nurse only. (It is important to be adequately chaperoned when discussing or examining for sexual health matters with anyone, but even more so with a child.) Most parents will see the value in your desire to explore confidential issues and if you are denied this opportunity, this raises the concern of possible child abuse. When you are able to discuss sexual health in a suitable environment, ask a full gynaecological history in an age-appropriate way.
Non-specific abdominal pain	This diagnosis of exclusion is made frequently in children but is poorly understood. It is usually less acute than other forms of abdominal pain in its onset. As a result, rather than causing parents to think that a child has appendicitis, it is the random and recurrent nature of the pain which causes much anxiety to the family. In order to diagnose non-specific abdominal pain, a child must be well and thriving in between episodes and other possible diagnoses must be excluded. Therefore the nature of the diagnosis usually requires outpatient referral to a paediatrician before it can be confirmed.
Inflammatory bowel disease	Crohn's disease and ulcerative colitis do occur, though uncommonly, in childhood. As well as abdominal pain, the children with inflammatory bowel disease usually present with bloody or mucousy diarrhoea. The features which set the children with inflammatory bowel disease apart from the more acute causes of bloody diarrhoea are the chronic signs and symptoms in the assessment. If a child has features suspicious for inflammatory bowel disease, they should be referred to the paediatric medical team.
Diabetic ketoacidosis	Especially when a child presents for the first time as a diabetic, this life-threatening condition can be easily missed in the hunt for a cause of abdominal pain. The child **can be mistakenly diagnosed as having a surgical abdomen** because there is abdominal pain and vomiting without diarrhoea in a patient who is significantly unwell. Because early recognition of this condition is essential to prevent the associated morbidity and mortality, it is worth including a blood sugar test in the initial assessment of any child with abdominal pain and vomiting. A urine dipstick will also point you towards the diagnosis but may not be immediately forthcoming. This condition should be managed according to local or national guidelines initially with cautious but adequate fluid resuscitation.

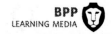

Diagnosis	Age group, common symptoms, etc.
Non accidental injury (NAI)	Child abuse can cause abdominal pain for physical or psychological reasons. When fever is absent and no other diagnosis is apparent, it is important to not just consider but also to exclude this possibility. This can only really be done by explaining that this is part of your job and ensuring that you have asked the child about physical and sexual abuse in a place and a way that would allow them to respond. This is a complicated but important subject which also has its own chapter (see Chapter 10).

Figure 6.1 Diagnoses for abdominal pain

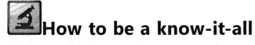How to be a know-it-all

Abdominal migraine is a cause of acute and recurrent abdominal pain which is probably under-diagnosed. If the specific questions are asked, there may be a history of headache, visual disturbance or nausea associated with the abdominal pains. A first degree relative with migraine also makes the diagnosis more likely. Identifying the diagnosis will often end months of wondering why the tummy pains are occurring. Treatment is the same as for migraine headaches, and both lack much evidence to support the standard treatments given.

De-mystifying the role of the paediatrician: what the paediatrician might do

One dilemma frequently faced by a referring doctor is 'who do I refer to?' If the provisional diagnosis is surgical, then surgeons who are skilled in managing the age group of child you are dealing with should be happy to take a direct referral.

Children with abdominal pain will frequently be admitted under the sole care or with the joint care of the paediatric medical team, especially in district general hospitals. The paediatrician is a good person to assess the child who has an uncertain diagnosis. They are also good at managing pain and fluid balance.

Ultimately if a child needs referring it is important to get them to the most appropriate specialist as quickly as possible. For example, a child with intussusception should be seen by a surgeon urgently, and if the doctor you speak to is unwilling, ask to speak to the consultant. However any doctor used to making referrals will know that sometimes surgeons are sceptical about our assessment. Although it may be frustrating for the paediatrician to be landed with a possible surgical problem it is in the best interest of the child that a willing doctor will admit the child to observe while managing their pain and fluid balance. If the paediatrician also assesses and feels that the problem is surgical then they can re-refer.

FAQs

Is it ok to give non-steroidal anti-inflammatory drugs (NSAIDS) to children who already have abdominal pain?

NSAIDs are useful analgesics for children but have well known side effects. There is a lack of evidence regarding the safety of NSAIDs when given to children who either have abdominal pain or an empty stomach. In practice, children seem to tolerate NSAIDs much better than adults do. I would advise a preference for giving paracetamol to any child who needed analgesia in any case. If this is not adequate then a NSAID may well improve pain control, so I use them cautiously.

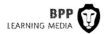

If used on an 'as required' basis for no more than a couple of days then gastritis is unusual. In fact, there can be a beneficial effect, since children who are febrile or have abdominal pain tend not to want to eat. If a NSAID can help to resolve these symptoms then they are more likely to feel like eating.

The notable exception to the rule is that **it is unwise to allow a child who is dehydrated to have NSAIDs.** Renal complications are also thankfully rare, but children with poor urine output are at greater risk and so should not take NSAIDs.

What do I tell the parents?

When I think that their child has colic:

"From what you have told me and having examined your baby, it seems most likely to me that the problem is colic. What we call colic is just the fact that the baby is feeling uncomfortable moving food around their bowels. No one really knows why some babies get this and others don't. The good news is that colic is completely harmless to your baby. The bad news is that nothing helps colic to go away."

"Colic does go away on its own after a few weeks, however in the meantime I understand how upsetting it is. Studies show that none of the medicines that you can buy for colic are any better than a placebo, so I do not use them. I understand that some parents feel that they work and I certainly have nothing against parents using them if that is the case. The most important thing to understand is that the colic will come and go as it pleases, so you should not exhaust yourself trying to make it go away. If you have made sure that your child is fed, warm, and in a clean nappy, then if they cry despite a cuddle, you are not doing anything wrong if you put them down in their cot. Sometimes a baby that cries constantly can be very frustrating and it is better to let them cry than to get upset with your baby."

When I think that the abdominal pain is most likely related to a viral illness and the child does not need to be referred to a surgeon:

"The tummy pain that your child has is probably due to the cold virus which they are suffering with at the moment. Everyone has glands inside their tummy just like the ones in the neck that get swollen when we are poorly. Children seem to be prone to getting painful swollen glands in their tummies when they are ill with any viral infection. Because that fits with what your child has at the moment and they are not worryingly unwell, I am happy for them to go home. They should respond well to medicines like paracetamol and they can have that at home just as easily. The tummy pain should start to go away as the cold/sore throat gets better, which might take a few days."

"I am always careful about tummy pain though, because it can be a little tricky sometimes. I don't think that your child has a problem like appendicitis, otherwise I would not think about suggesting that you take them home. However, if the pain gets worse despite medicines, or your child starts vomiting, stops drinking or seems more unwell, it is best to get them seen again. At any point, if you think that something has changed and you are worried, I want you to bring your child back."

Flowchart for assessing the child with abdominal pain

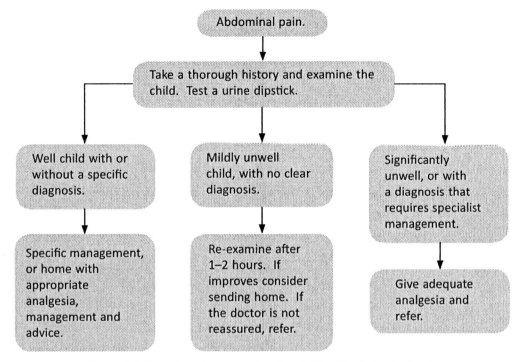

Figure 6.2 Flowchart for assessing the child with abdominal pain

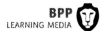 ## Summary for abdominal pain

- The causes of abdominal pain in children are multiple. Most are not harmful, however, abdominal pain can be a symptom of serious illness.
- The diagnosis is usually apparent from the history, and should be supported by careful examination.
- A urine specimen should usually be tested.
- In most cases a cause is suspected and the child is well enough to be allowed home, but appropriate advice is essential to ensure that the child returns if more unwell.

If a child is unwell, or there is doubt, it is best to seek a second opinion from a colleague either in your workplace or in secondary care.

Chapter 7
Funny turns

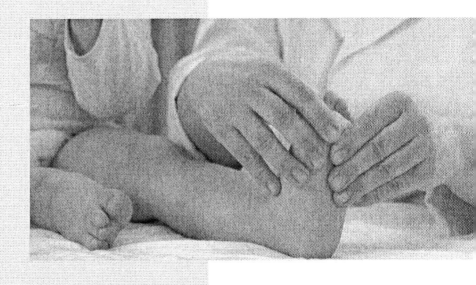

Funny turns

Background

- One of the most common reasons for a child to present for assessment is that they have recently had an event of some kind. This could be any one of a huge number of witnessed phenomena and the child may be well or unwell at presentation.
- Funny turns include colour changes, unresponsive episodes and abnormal movements of various descriptions.
- Children may present as an urgent case but may also come days or even weeks later if the child seemed completely well immediately after the event.

Usually, after a funny turn of some kind, the adult who witnessed the event is very concerned about the cause of the funny turn. As the assessing clinician, your job is to address these anxieties and also to obtain as thorough a history as possible in order to make a decision about whether you are yourself concerned. To make such an assessment it is important to have a good working knowledge of the various funny turn's that occur in childhood, when they are likely to occur and what their significance is.

How to assess

Of course, if a child appears ill, then early examination and management of ABC are the first priority. However if a diagnosis is made regarding a funny turn, it is usually through the history. Time spent getting a good eye-witness account of what happened will be far more likely to give you useful information than a full neurological examination. Neurological examination is also valuable yet often difficult to interpret.

- What was the child like before the event? Were they well? Had they been their usual selves? Did something seem to set it off?
- Ask about head injuries and recent illnesses.
- What happened? Ask for specifics about what is meant by everything.
- Was there a colour change? If so then what colour? Ask the parents to show you an example if possible.
- Were there any abnormal movements? What were they? Ask the parents to show you. If they can't do that then I usually show them what a shiver looks like, what uncoordinated flailing looks like and what clonic jerking looks like so they can tell me if it was one of those.
- How long did it last for? Be politely sceptical about the answer to this question. When you think something terrible is happening to your child then seconds really do seem like minutes. Try counting out ten to twenty seconds and asking if it lasted longer than that.
- Was the child truly unresponsive during the event? People often say unresponsive when they mean less responsive. What did they do to assess responsiveness?
- Have there been any funny turns in the past?
- Ask about development.
- Ask about family history of funny turns.

Conducting a neurological assessment in a child is as much about observation as it is about actually physically examining the child. At the risk of encouraging brevity, I would suggest that most of your neurological examination is complete the minute that you lay eyes on the child. It is sometimes difficult to know exactly how to describe a child's neurological state, but you will usually know whether you are concerned within the first few seconds. Below

 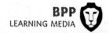

are some specific questions which you should try to answer.

- Are they alert? (see altered consciousness in the terminology section)
- If alert, then are they subdued or interested in their surroundings? Is there eye contact?
- Does the child smile? If so then the likelihood of any significant neurological deficit is very small.
- Do they seem lethargic or are they active?
- If sitting or lying then check tone. There is little point in this context checking tone in a child who is active.
- Are facial movements symmetrical?

While it is possible to write a full page in the notes about a detailed neurological examination for a child who, for example, had an episode of unresponsiveness and jerking movements, I think that for an initial assessment there is no real need to put too much detail if you feel that the child is normal. If I write: 'Alert and smiling. Playing and chatty. Walking and using both arms equally', then is anything really added by listing tendon reflexes and a cranial nerve examination?

A guide to the common specific diagnoses at different ages

After your assessment you may or may not be able to make a diagnosis. It is usually possible to have a reasonable amount of certainty about what happened to the child and tests rarely add to this. Below are tables of common causes of funny turns through the different ages of childhood, including those that would be considered normal physiological events. I have also included rarer causes of funny turns where these are important diagnoses to make.

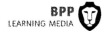

Babies (from birth to twelve months)

Diagnosis	Clinical picture
Benign sleep myoclonus	This consists of sudden and often repetitive jerking movements in an otherwise well and normally developing child. This is a phenomenon that almost all babies exhibit and the movements are simply involuntary movements associated with sleep. Some babies do this more than others. Some parents find these quite alarming and worry that their child is having 'fits'. The child is of course well, thriving and developing normally. **The movements are always during sleep or as sleep is starting or finishing.** If the movements are repetitive they can be subdued easily by holding the limb. Reassurance and safety-netting is all that is required in these cases.
Apparent life-threatening episodes (ALTE)	This is not a diagnosis but rather a declaration of concern about an event in a child under the age of twelve months. Any event such as a brief apnoea, floppy episode or cause for alarm that is not clearly explained by a benign cause (eg. choked on some milk and is now fine) is usually described as an ALTE. **If a baby has a floppy episode or changes colour then this may be an indicator of a significant underlying illness.** The child may have sepsis or any number of less common but also life-threatening illnesses. The explanation may also be something more benign such as gastro-oesophageal reflux. One concern is that an unexplained ALTE may precede sudden infant death (SID), though no link has ever been proven. For all these reasons, whenever a child under the age of one presents with an event that is neither benign nor easily explained by benign phenomena it is usual to refer for observation and assessment by the paediatric team.
Infantile spasms (West's syndrome)	This is an epilepsy syndrome which usually occurs in the first few months of life. It is **progressive and affects development.** However, since **early treatment improves outcome**, recognition of this rare condition is important. The usual scenario is one of flexor spasms of both the upper limbs (and sometimes the legs as well), which project forwards every few seconds. These spasms usually occur in clusters. They occur while awake or asleep and in between clusters the child often seems well. If you see a child who you suspect of having infantile spasms they should be referred urgently for assessment and not just as an outpatient. It is essential to take a good history to detect conditions such as this, including development, and examine well before assuming that the parents are describing benign sleep myoclonus.
Gastro-oesophageal reflux disease (GORD)	**Gastro-oesophageal reflux is a common cause of funny turns in babies.** They can go floppy, go pale, arch their back and may not have any obvious reflux or choking. Since any of these symptoms may be associated with more dangerous conditions, this presumptive diagnosis should be made only in the context of considering other causes and while keeping an open mind after making a provisional diagnosis. If the clinical scenario best fits reflux and the child is otherwise well then a trial of antacids would be a reasonable approach as long as the baby was reviewed to ensure that the problem had resolved after a week.

Figure 7.1 Diagnoses of funny turns in babies (from birth to twelve months)

Preschool age (twelve months to five years)

Diagnosis	Clinical picture
Febrile convulsions	This is the phenomenon of epileptic-type seizures associated with febrile illness in a child who is otherwise neurologically and developmentally normal. The reasons why some children get febrile convulsions are not really understood, however, those that do often get them repeatedly with recurrent illnesses. **Most will just occur as a single event** and not otherwise affect the child. The history should be one of a normal child having an epileptic seizure (usually generalised and tonic-clonic) at the same time as or just before a fever. Note that an idiopathic epileptic seizure can raise temperature, so evidence of some kind of illness is also important. The management is that of a good explanation and the treatment of whatever illness is associated. There is actually very little evidence that aggressive anti-fever treatment prevents further seizures but fever should be managed for its own reasons. Most importantly, if a child has had a fever and a seizure they should be observed until they are convincingly recovered to the extent that you can be sure that they do not have meningitis or encephalitis. Any focal element to the seizure, or a prolonged seizure (greater than five minutes) should make the clinician even more suspicious of intracranial infection, including abscess. Febrile convulsions do not usually occur in children under five months, so be very wary of diagnosing this in babies.
Reflex anoxic seizures/spells	These rather alarming events occur mainly in this age group. The usual story is of a child who has an **unexpected and often painful stimulus** (eg runs into something) or gets a fright or gets upset. For those children who are prone to reflex anoxic seizures this stimulus triggers a vasovagal reaction with or without a full blown epileptic-type of convulsion. The child will usually go 'deathly white' and collapse. They may or may not convulse for a few seconds before recovering. The diagnosis is made based on the classic history without the need for tests. The management is that of explanation, advice about keeping a child safe during a seizure and the assurance that the child will one day outgrow the tendency to do this.
Breath-holding attacks	These are similar to reflex anoxic seizures but are more associated with tantrums and upsets. There may be some behavioural element to these episodes. Usually the child screams and then stops breathing or seems to hold their breath. As a result they usually go blue before collapsing. As with reflex anoxic attacks there may be progression to a convulsion. Again, the child grows out of this tendency.
Rigors	A rigor is a transient cardiovascular collapse, with unresponsiveness associated with an infection of some kind. They are dramatic events and having seen both rigors and febrile convulsions, I can understand why parents always rush their child in after a rigor but occasionally see a GP a few days after a febrile convulsion. Rigors are one of the most difficult things to differentiate from febrile convulsions in this age group. I have frequently heard parents give the same description of an episode to two paediatricians and had one decide that the episode was a rigor and the other diagnose a febrile convulsion. Rigors cause floppiness, unresponsiveness, abnormal movements and colour change just as febrile convulsions do. The fact that the movement during a rigor is more of a shiver, and during a seizure it is classically rhythmic jerking, doesn't always

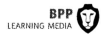

Diagnosis	Clinical picture
Rigors	help. Parents are so anxious after either that they often say yes to both having occurred. In many ways however it does not matter too much which has occurred. The management of a child who has had a rigor is to establish what the underlying infection is and treat it. **Either a rigor or a febrile convulsion should compel the doctor to eliminate meningitis and other significant infections.** Since rigors are particularly associated with urinary tract infections (UTIs) you should usually get a good urine specimen following a rigor.

Figure 7.2 Diagnoses of funny turns in preschool (from twelve months to five years)

School age (five to eighteen years)

Diagnosis	Clinical picture
Vasovagal episodes	**Faints of all kinds become quite common in school age children and especially adolescents.** Although they may be related to underlying anaemia, vasovagal episodes often defy explanation. The classic history is that of a sensation of feeling nauseous or hot just before losing vision. People often recall a blacking out during which time they could still hear voices. Witnesses usually describe the person going pale and then slumping to the floor. Recovery is variable and often prolonged by embarrassment. Vasovagal episodes are worth investigating with a full blood count (FBC) and an electrocardiogram (ECG). A lying down and standing blood pressure is also a useful test.
Absences vs. inattention	By their nature children have variable attention spans and so often appear to be having absence episodes. They will not be aware of having absence seizures so making the diagnosis can be difficult. Classically **the child with absence seizures will have these events at home and at school and during any activity,** while inattention is often limited to certain activities such as French lessons. There may also be a sudden drop in the child's school performance after the onset of absence seizures. Absence seizures are one condition for which electroencephalograms (EEGs) can make the diagnosis as long as the clinician who requests it understands the test and how to interpret the result.
The epilepsies	Idiopathic unprovoked epileptic seizures can occur at any age but become more common as childhood progresses. When a classic tonic-clonic generalised seizure is witnessed then it is appropriate to refer the child for further assessment. However it is usually inappropriate to start treatment at this stage. Many seizures will not recur and anti-epileptic treatment will not actually improve the long term outcome for the child. Anti-epileptic drugs will hopefully reduce seizure frequency, but a pattern rather than a one-off event is needed before deciding to start treatment.

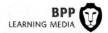

Diagnosis	Clinical picture
Migraine	Migraine without aura (intense, often unilateral headaches) rarely present as acute events. More likely to present urgently are migraines with aura, events with various possible symptoms which can cause them to mimic other illnesses. The headache may be associated with nausea, vomiting, visual disturbances and even peripheral neurological symptoms such as numbness and weakness. **Migraines may be mistaken for meningitis, strokes, and sub-arachnoid haemorrhage.** A family or past medical history of classic or hemiplegic migraine (now classified as migraine with aura) makes the diagnosis of migraine more likely. Usually the diagnosis is made on the basis of a classic history (prodrome of nausea or dizziness, visual disturbances such as scotoma or tunnel vision and headache) and the absence of persistent neurological findings on examination. If in doubt I think that these cases cause enough anxiety to warrant discussion with a colleague.
Non-epileptic seizures	For reasons that are poorly understood, a proportion of adolescents will have what may be quite convincingly convulsions, yet are non-epileptic (including those that would previously have been termed pseudo-seizures). The important thing is to be aware of this as a possibility and to avoid writing these off as attention seeking. A psychological and social history from these children is essential to identify any underlying stresses.
Substance misuse	One possible reason for an unexplained presentation with abnormal neurological signs or symptoms is ingestion of some kind. In order to diagnose this, a good history is required, including what medicines are available at home and what the child has been doing prior to presentation. Substance misuse is most commonly missed in younger children (age 10–13) because as doctors we are reluctant to think of children taking such drugs.

Figure 7.3 Diagnoses of funny turns in school age (five to eighteen years)

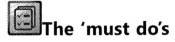 ## The 'must do's

 ## Pitfalls to avoid

The 'must do's	Pitfalls to avoid
☑ First assess whether the child is well before trying to obtain a detailed history ☑ If unwell assess airway, breathing and circulation (ABC), consciousness level and **don't forget to check a blood sugar level** ☑ Obtain a detailed first hand account of the event from the child if possible and at least one eyewitness ☑ Make detailed notes of the history	☒ Don't rely on people's *assessment* of what happened. If they tell you the child had a fit, ask them to describe what happened. ☒ Don't rely on tests to make a diagnosis. Investigations after a funny turn should add to a diagnosis but do not make the diagnosis. ☒ It is important to consider non-accidental injury when there is a child presenting with an apparently unexplained funny turn. ☒ Don't forget to consider factitious illness and drugs.

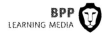

How to be a know-it-all

- **It is better to avoid making a diagnosis than to make the wrong one.** If a child might have had a rigor or a febrile convulsion, leave the diagnosis open and describe what happened. It is bad practice to put terms like 'fit' into the notes. Was it a fit of laughter? Instead either write what happened or a clear medical term such as 'isolated generalised tonic-clonic convulsion with no focal features lasting 1–2 minutes'.
- **It is useful to have an idea of normal development** so that you can make a quick assessment of whether a child's previous development is normal.

While there are much more specific assessment tools available, these are impractical for most consultations. The following quick reference guide is the rough guide which I use to make a preliminary assessment. I start by asking if the child has reached the average milestone for their age. If the answer is no, then I work backwards until I find a milestone which they have reached. If they say yes then you can just leave it at that. To make a more complete assessment, you should also ask about social and behavioural development and enquire about hearing and vision. However, asking about motor and verbal development tends to work quickly and has a good pick-up rate for any developmental problems.

Age	Motor	Verbal
Six months	Can roll over. Can hold things in one hand.	Makes some noises.
Twelve months	Can sit unsupported. Can crawl or bottom shuffle. Can cruise around furniture and may be able to walk.	Has babbled and should now be making some recognisable words eg 'dada'.
Eighteen months	Can walk without help.	Makes several recognisable words.
Two years	Can go up stairs with help. Can kick a ball.	Puts two words together eg 'want that', 'more chocolate'.
Three years	Can go up stairs without help. Can jump.	Makes more complex sentences. Should be mostly understandable by a stranger.
Four to five years	Can throw and sometimes catch a ball. Can draw a person.	Should speak in full sentences and be fully understandable.

Figure 7.4 A quick guide to developmental milestones

Also worth knowing

- **Electoencephalograms (EEGs) are not nearly as helpful as one would hope** when assessing children who have had funny turns. They can confuse matters to such an extent that I believe that only paediatricians should be requesting them. EEGs are reported as normal in half of the children who do have seizures. Likewise, about one in ten children who have no tendency to epileptic seizures will have some vague 'abnormality' on an EEG. This makes the EEG a very poor screening test even if only used for children who have had a funny turn. It is far better to make a diagnosis based on the history than allow an EEG to sway an uncertain diagnosis. So be confident that EEGs are best requested *after* a diagnosis is made rather than making the diagnosis in the first place.

- Lying down and standing blood pressures are often taken incorrectly and can be misleading. It is essential to take the baseline blood pressure after lying down for five minutes with the correctly sized cuff at the level of the heart. Then the patient should stand up and be measured after one minute and three minutes. This is time consuming, but laying a patient down, checking their blood pressure quickly, standing them up and doing it again does not give useful information. If taken time and done properly then a systolic drop of 20mm Hg (mercury) is significant.

- Remember to consider that both epileptic and non-epileptic seizures may be related to substance misuse.

De-mystifying the role of the paediatrician: what the paediatrician might do

After an acute presentation the involvement of a paediatrician will depend greatly on the condition of the child. Children who have made a complete recovery following an episode that did not seem life-threatening may be just discussed or referred non-urgently.

If the child has not made a complete recovery or the episode itself was concerning then in most cases a paediatrician would prefer to see the child acutely. Following their own assessment, the paediatrician can decide whether to observe, investigate or even treat, for example if infections are suspected.

FAQs

Was this a febrile convulsion or a rigor?

The simple answer is that it doesn't matter as much as you might think. In both cases the abnormal episode is symptomatic of an underlying infection. The focus of the infection is more important than the event which it caused. If the infection is benign and the child has made a full recovery, then uncertainty about the event is secondary.

Both febrile convulsions and rigors produce altered consciousness and abnormal movements. I do not believe that there is a list of symptoms that can distinguish easily between them. The only way that I am ever completely sure is when I am convinced of true repeated clonic jerking in the history. In the absence of a clear history of fitting, the diagnosis often remains uncertain. In such circumstances it is reasonable to explain that the child might have had a febrile convulsion. However the implications of having a febrile fit are not as significant as the issue of being certain that there is no serious infection underlying the funny turn.

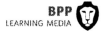

What do I tell the parents?

When I believe that their child has had a febrile convulsion:

"The thing that affected your child earlier is called a febrile fit, or a fit due to a fever. A lot of children are affected by these in their pre-school years. The important thing is that your child has made a good recovery after having this fit."

"Having a febrile fit does not mean that your child has epilepsy. Most of these fits are one-offs although some children do go on to have further episodes when they have other infections.

We expect those children to grow out of that tendency by the time they are about six years old."

"In most cases febrile fits will last less than five minutes and will not be dangerous. They do not usually need treatment. You cannot necessarily prevent them and all that we advise is to do your best to control your child's fever when they are ill just as you would do normally."

"Because we do not expect this to affect your child in the long term, we do not need to follow them up. If an episode happens again we will see your child at the time and reassess the situation then."

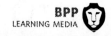

Flowchart for assessing the child with funny turns

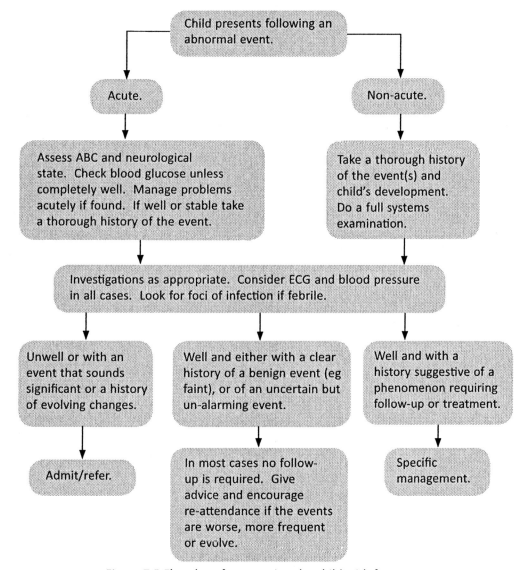

Figure 7.5 Flowchart for assessing the child with funny turns

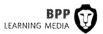Summary for funny turns

- Events which might occur in childhood include neurological, cardiovascular, behavioural, physiological and psychological phenomena.
- A good and thorough history is required to make a clear diagnosis.
- If the diagnosis is unclear then it is best to keep the diagnosis open than to make an incorrect diagnosis.
- If there is doubt about a diagnosis then tests may cause more confusion.

Chapter 8
Constipation

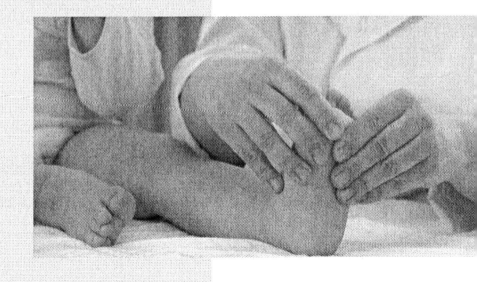

Constipation

Background

Although this might seem like a strange condition to dedicate an entire chapter to, constipation is a common problem in childhood, and often underlies unexplained symptoms in children. Every child has a different bowel habit to the next child, so knowing whether a child is constipated is often difficult, and when you add this to the unreliability of reported bowel habit, it is easy to see how inadequate passage of stools can be easily missed.

It is commonly believed that children who become constipated eat mainly 'junk food', which is low in fibre, and that children who eat healthily have normal bowel habits. Experience demonstrates though that **any child can become constipated** and that **most of these children do not usually have a clearly identifiable 'reason'.** Most children who become constipated do so apparently without a cause or underlying pathology.

To take an adequate history, one must first have a working definition of constipation. One possible definition is that **constipation is the failure to pass stools in a physiologically adequate way, leading to adverse symptoms.** The normal physiology is for the large bowel to produce formed stools, and for the rectum to evacuate these as soon as the rectum contains stool. Children who become constipated have a failure in that process, which may be due to poor diet, poor fluid intake or an underlying medical condition. The processes governing opening ones bowels are complicated and the psychological/behavioural aspect to constipation is essential to understand.

When we are born, stool passage is a reflex neurological phenomenon. The fact that well babies can get constipated shows that this process can fail. Later in life we impose higher control over the function of our anal sphincter. It is therefore possible to override the desire to pass stool when higher control is learned and this ability can contribute to the development of constipation. Children will not open their bowels for a variety of reasons. They may simply withhold stools because they are too busy to go to the toilet; they have block towers to build and games to play. Often in constipation a vicious cycle develops because the hard stool causes anal discomfort and so the child is reluctant to go to pass stool for fear of pain. In fact, any negative association with going to the toilet, including criticism for soiling, can contribute to a child's constipation problem.

It is also important to understand the impact that constipation in children has on the child and their families, especially in school age children. The effect on the family dynamic is often considerable and the daily attention given to the problem makes it into an anxiety of elephant proportions. The child's self esteem and confidence is also affected. Child and parent alike end up feeling that they are failures. Your job is to turn this around.

How to assess

The first thing to realise is that **many children with constipation do not present with constipation as such.** Some parents will express a concern that their child is not going to the toilet properly. Perversely, these children may well have normal bowel habit, and a parent or carer who expects a different pattern of passing stools for some reason. Some children who present with a concern about bowel habit are truly constipated. The ways that constipation presents are many and varied including:

- Diarrhoea
- Abdominal pains
- Urinary frequency

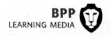

- Urinary tract infection
- Soiling
- Poor weight gain
- Anaemia
- Anorexia

The key to diagnosing constipation lies in thinking of it as a possibility and then asking the right questions. Examination may not be as helpful as you would hope, so a good history is essential.

- How often does the child open their bowels?
- How big a stool do they pass? Do they pass any small amounts between stools?
- What does the stool look like? This can be subjective, but essentially you want to know if it looks like animal droppings, a sausage or sloppy curry.
- Are they still in nappies?
- Do they soil?
- Have they always had this problem? If it has recently appeared, then what happened around that time? Was there a change in diet for example or an emotional upset?
- Ask about the specifics of diet and fluid intake.
- Ask about abdominal pain and its association with meal times and opening bowels.
- Ask about anal pain and bleeding.
- Ask about urinary symptoms and past urine infections.
- Ask about medications and family history of bowel disorders.
- Ask about past and present emotional upsets.

When examining the child, look for:

- General wellbeing, conjunctival pallor.
- Weigh the child and plot the result in their hand held record or a growth chart, and compare the total to previous weights.
- Abdominal distension.
- Abdominal tenderness and masses. (Faeces may be palpable, but not always easily.

Sometimes they are soft, and so therefore difficult to feel. A fullness of the left lower quadrant is suspicious for constipation.)
- Examine the anus externally (*do not perform a rectal examination*), looking for soiling and fissures.

The 'must do's

☑ Be specific about the history of the bowel habit. Do not accept the answer that it is 'normal'. Find out how often and what the child is passing.

☑ Get details about diet. The only way to adequately do this is to ask what the child has actually eaten and drunk in the past 24 hours, hour by hour.

☑ Remember that trauma to the anus can be sexual abuse which itself can lead to constipation. Without other causes for concern, the anal fissure can be explained by the constipation; however, if there are other features which lead you to suspect abuse, include the constipation and anal fissure among these suspicious features.

Pitfalls to avoid

Avoid under-treating or partially treating constipation. By the time that they present for a medical assessment, children usually have well established constipation that requires adequate treatment for many weeks or months. Short bursts of laxatives temporarily improve things if you are lucky but may make matters worse and cause the family to lose faith in the treatment when the problem comes back. Do not be fooled by the fact that the child or parents have only been aware of symptoms for a short period. By the time things are bad enough to seek help, no minor intervention is likely to work.

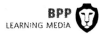

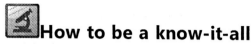

How to be a know-it-all

The best way to be a bit clever about constipation is to diagnose it in a child with vague symptoms. At some point in your career you will see a child with weight loss, or abdominal pain or urinary symptoms and you will think, 'I wonder if this could all be due to constipation?' Ask a little bit about bowel habit and you may find that you are the first person who went into any detail. If you are the person who finally identifies the cause for a child's symptoms you will find that the parents are very impressed.

A guide to the management of constipation

The management of children under one year old is a rather different matter to that of the older child. **Babies can often go through periods of days where no stools are passed.** If they are asymptomatic then they are best managed by adding water to their intake, and ensuring this is offered between feeds and not before a feed so that the child still gets the calories that they need. If the baby seems to be getting distressed by the constipation, then a glycerine suppository as well as water may allow the child to pass a stool and help to get things moving. The size of this will depend on the size of the baby. The current British National Formulary for Children (BNFc) recommends a 1mg suppository between the ages of one month and one year. Before one month, suppositories are rarely needed. If you do need to use glycerine, you will often need to repeat the dose.

Fruit juice has also been traditionally recommended. Some advise fresh orange juice and some recommend prune juice. There is in fact very little evidence that these are effective or indeed as to how they work if they do work. It may be that any laxative effect is due to poorly absorbed sugars in the fruit juice rather than a fibre effect as most would assume. Since giving water is just as lacking in evidence but is presumably less likely to do harm, I would recommend a preference for simple water (sterile water for babies) in the first place.

The wonderful thing about treating constipation in older children is that anyone can do it if they have the confidence and they are willing to spend the time. Even if you are only seeing the child as a one-off, such as in the emergency department, or an out-of-hours GP service, it is possible to make a real difference to what is a long term problem which has a huge impact on families.

Education and advice

The first stage of treatment is explanation. Understand that 'constipation' will not adequately explain the problem. Enthusiastic explanations of how our bowels are supposed to work and a description of what happens when things go wrong are vital to getting the child and parents on board for the necessary changes which will hopefully resolve the problem. I find that **pictures are useful** and some ready made pictures are available from various sources. However, because I am not that well organised, I usually draw my own (see figure 8.1).

At the end of your explanation, the parents (and child if old enough) should understand the following:

- Constipation happens commonly in childhood, and usually for no particular reason.
- **The problem is usually there for many weeks or months before anyone realises that this is what is going on,** so it is unlikely that the problem will go away on its own.
- Usually, poo moves through the tubes in the tummy and when it gets to the end of the tube we feel it there and push it out into the toilet.
- When we get constipated, there is poo that is not coming out when it should.

- This poo stretches the tubes, making the muscles in the tummy weak, and numbing the nerves which are supposed to tell you when to poo.
- There are lots of things that can be done to make this all better but it will need you to work hard to make it better.
- It may take just as long for you to get better as it took for the problem to sneak up, so this will take several months to get it properly better. Remember the stretched muscles and nerves that I told you about: they need time to get their strength back.

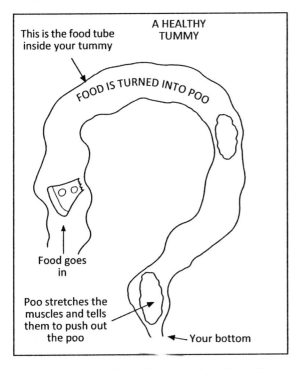

Figure 8.1 Normal bowels: an explanation of how bowels usually function

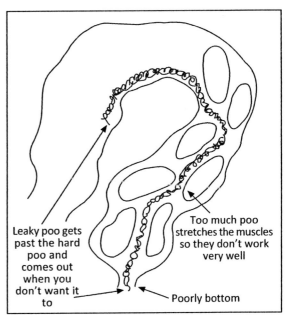

Figure 8.2 Constipation: an explanation of what happens when bowels are constipated and why there can be overflow diarrhoea

Hopefully, you will now have a captive audience who understand the problem and are eagerly awaiting your advice. There is a lot of advice to give but don't let that put you off. It is the simple things which make the most difference in the long term, even if they do need medication in the medium term. **Good advice is important, and should be repeated at each visit, as it is quickly forgotten.** Also, if it is emphasised at each contact with a health professional, the family will better appreciate the sincerity of this advice. If possible, write it down and ask the child to repeat back to you what the important bits were. The key points are:

- Even if diet may not be to blame (this is important to emphasise because no parent believes that they feed their child poorly, so by implying that they do, you have immediately lost your rapport), there are certain things that help constipation get better and some things that make it worse. **Bad foods for constipation include chocolate, crisps,**

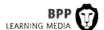

131

sweets, biscuits and cakes. Good foods are fruit and vegetables and cereals with lots of fibre in them. Unfortunately you have to eat the good foods, and get rid of the bad foods.

- Drinking water is also important. Milk is healthy for bones, however drinking nothing but milk can make you constipated. Sugary and fizzy drinks are very bad for constipation. Pure orange juice can help a little bit, but nothing is as good as drinking lots and lots and lots of water.

- Because the nerves are not working as well as they should, they don't always send the message that you need a poo. But, **when you have just had a meal, your body gives out a chemical that makes the muscles in your tummy stronger.** So the best thing to do is for the child to sit on the toilet for at least five minutes after every meal. Encourage the child to do a poo but tell them not to become upset if they don't. The more a child spends trying after meals, the sooner the nerves will work again.

- Because the muscles are all stretched and weak, this problem usually needs help to begin with to get better. The medication that we use makes the muscles stronger, and keeps the bowels empty enough to get their strength back. Because this takes time, children usually need to take the medicine for a few months. If the child stops the medicine as soon as it has started working, the muscles are still weak and the problem quickly comes back.

Medication

The issue of medication is seemingly a thorny one. There is a belief that use of laxatives creates dependence. I believe that this misconception exists for two reasons. Firstly, laxatives only temporarily improve bowel function. If therefore the problem is not a temporary one, the problem returns on stopping the medication. Secondly, medication is stopped too soon too often so that the child has little hope of good bowel function.

Both situations give the impression that the child has become dependent.

The solution is to **treat for long enough to allow good bowel function to develop**, and at the same time, ensure all that can be done is done to ensure that long term, pro-constipation factors such as poor diet, fluid intake and bowel habit are removed from the equation.

The issue of which medication to use is a matter of personal preference:

- Glycerine suppositories are best used in the children under one year old. They work by lubricating the area where they dissolve, so make little or no difference to a child with proper constipation. However the effect that they have is slightly greater for very small children and using glycerine may avoid the need for other medication.

- **Medications such as lactulose have a place but should rarely be used.** Lactulose is a sugar which works as an osmotic, making the resulting stools softer. As a sugar, it causes tooth decay and as an osmotic agent it can further dehydrate children who may not be drinking adequately. Additionally, where there is overflow or soiling, the softening of the stools will make this worse.

- **A stimulant is almost always needed to help the bowels to clear the large hard stools which are causing so much of a problem.** The choice of stimulant will depend on what you or your department are used to. I have seen a great deal of success with macrogol powders (eg Movicol) in recent years and find that they are generally effective and well tolerated. Whenever prescribing a stimulant laxative, you should advise two things. Firstly, that this will probably be needed for several months. Secondly, after starting the medicine, there may be a worsening of tummy pain and incontinence. This is because the muscles are starting to work again. It is therefore a good idea to avoid school time when starting stimulant laxatives. Usually this effect only lasts a couple of days. The aim after any initial 'clear out' is to give adequate doses of enough stimulant laxative to allow them to easily pass a soft, well-formed stool on most days. This needs to be continued as long as it is needed. Eventually, as tone and sensation improve, the child should find themselves over-medicated and wean themselves off.

Now this needs to be followed up. If the child has been seen in the out-of-hours GP service or emergency department then the next step is probably to get the parents to book the child an appointment with their own GP. Ideally they will need something in writing to take with them to make sure that the doctor who sees them understands your plan. They can then decide whether they feel equipped to follow through with the management of the constipation, or refer to a paediatrician for ongoing care.

De-mystifying the role of the paediatrician: what the paediatrician might do

Children can be referred to a paediatrician at any point for help with managing their constipation. Even so, most children are managed without tests or prescribing medications which are not licenced for use with children. Most of what the doctor does in the paediatric clinic can be done by any doctor who follows the management guidelines stated previously.

Occasionally children will have investigations, but this is the exception rather than the rule. Children should probably be referred for assessment if they remain on medication for more than six months or if they do not improve despite moderate doses of stimulant laxatives.

The services of a nurse specialist may be available in secondary care. Because constipation is such a common and persistent problem in child health, many trusts employ a nurse with a special interest in managing constipation. These nurse specialists are a valuable resource and can spend more time explaining the problem and treatment, as well as being a contact point for the family when needed.

FAQs

How long does constipation need to be treated for?

I was taught in medical school that using laxatives for prolonged periods leads the bowel to become dependent on treatment in order to work. In fact, I don't believe that there is any evidence that prescribing laxatives somehow causes the bowel to forget how to work. The reason why people become constipated after stopping laxatives is that whatever caused them to become constipated in the first place (whether dietary, behavioural or pathological) is still there, causing the problem to recur. Imagine if we applied the same approach to conditions such as diabetes and stopped medication early for fear of tolerance!

I believe that a good rule of thumb is to **assume that your patient will need treatment to be given for as long as they have had constipation,** including all the time that they didn't realise that this was the case (you can usually deduce this from the history, from the onset of related symptoms such as abdominal pain or reduced appetite). Usually this means months rather than weeks of treatment. I believe treatment is needed for this long because it takes a long time to reach the point where bowels are functioning so poorly that people will seek medical attention. It will therefore take a long time to restore normal function.

What do I tell the parents?

When I have said that I think that their child is constipated, and they say that this is impossible because their child does poo sometimes:

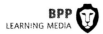

"Constipation is to do with what is stuck inside rather than what comes out. Often, children who are constipated do poo but not enough is coming out properly to keep things as empty as they need to be, to keep the bowels healthy. I like to think of this as a bit like traffic jams. Imagine that you are in a traffic jam that takes you an hour just to get to a set of traffic lights. If you are a pedestrian stood at the traffic lights, you will see lots of cars coming through, but there is still a mile long queue of cars. Constipation is like this. Some poo is coming out but it is what is waiting to come out which causes the problem."

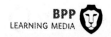

Flowchart for assessing the child with constipation

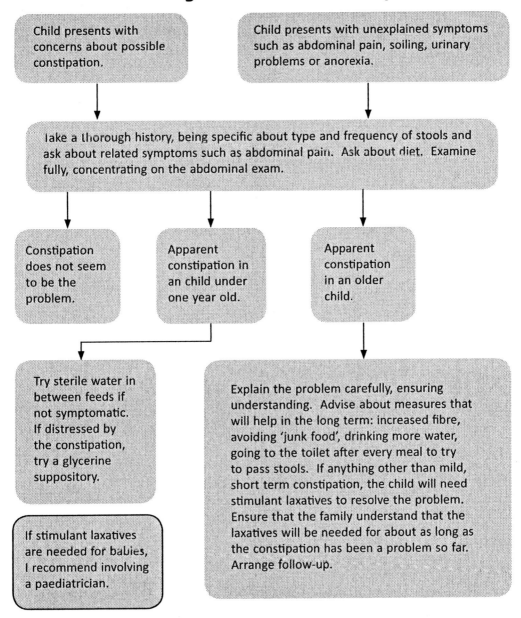

Figure 8.3 Flowchart for assessing the child with constipation

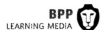

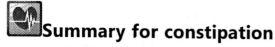

Summary for constipation

- Constipation is a common, often unrecognised problem in children, and causes significant long term problems to the children who are affected as well as their families.
- Most constipation is not due to an underlying cause, and in the majority of cases, children can be managed in general practice without need for investigations.
- The key to treating the child with significant constipation is to give adequate doses of enough stimulant laxative to allow them to easily pass a soft, well-formed stool on most days. This needs to be continued as long as it is needed.
- All children with constipation need to understand the problem and the treatment. Child and family alike need to be motivated to ensure good diet, good fluid intake and good bowel habit.
- Every clinical contact with a child who has constipation is an opportunity to check that everything is being done to optimise diet, fluid intake, bowel habit and exercise, and that this is fully understood and implemented.

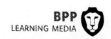

Chapter 9
The child with diarrhoea and/ or vomiting

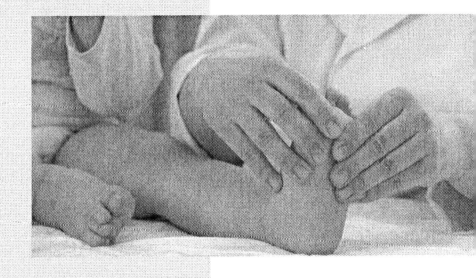

The child with diarrhoea and/or vomiting

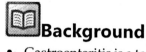

Background

- Gastroenteritis is a term used to describe the illness when children present with a vomiting and diarrhoeal illness of presumed infectious origin.
- Such illness is very common in any age, but especially in children who are younger (because they still have a naive immune system), and children who are exposed to lots of other children at home, school or indeed in hospital.
- The vast majority of gastroenteritis in children is managed by families without seeking medical intervention.
- Despite the fact that diarrhoeal illnesses are still the biggest killers of children in the developing world, only about one in every one hundred cases do children in the developed world even get admitted to hospital.
- Deaths in developed countries are extremely rare.
- Gastroenteritis can cause children to be very ill indeed but regardless of the severity of the illness, parental anxiety often runs high. I blame this on the parental instinct to feed children and to keep children well, both of which are of course frustrated by the child with diarrhoea and vomiting.

Most children who present with gastroenteritis will be essentially well. Often, the diarrhoea is the more prominent feature and the child is taking good amounts of fluid to compensate. Even when there is vomiting, children seem to manage to keep enough fluids down and compensate in other ways, such that they do cope until the illness burns out.

However, do not be too easily reassured. Those children who do run into trouble with gastroenteritis have reached the end of their ability to cope. They have moved fluid from the intracellular compartment until they have no further ability to do so, they have burnt up all their energy reserves and they have ratcheted up their cardiovascular compensatory mechanisms so that there is nowhere left to go. As a result, when they pass the point of coping, they become quite suddenly and catastrophically unwell.

Fear not though, with careful assessment and good management, success is virtually guaranteed. The odds are very much on the side of the child getting better. Your job is to help them to do this for themselves and identify the children who are not getting better, and cannot get better.

How to assess

Although a history in the context of gastroenteritis does not have to be extensive, there are some important facts to elicit:

- How long has the child been unwell?
- Is there diarrhoea, vomiting or both? Which appeared first?
- Is the child drinking? How much do the parents think the child has had today?
- Is the child passing urine? How many times today?
- Has there been any blood or mucous in the stool? Any blood or bile in the vomit?
- Have there been any floppy or unresponsive episodes at home?
- Is anyone else unwell?
- Has there been any foreign travel?
- Now, before you examine the child, put on some gloves. (The last thing you want is to get a tummy bug in the week before you are due to go on holiday.)
- Look at the child's overall health. Do they look well, a bit unwell or quite unwell?
- Note the child's colour and facial appearance. Are they pale? Are the eyes sunken into dark sockets? Is the skin turgor normal?

- Look for wet mucous membranes. Dry lips are an unhelpful sign, especially when a child has been crying, but dry eyes and mouth are significant.
- Check the pulse, and check the capillary refill over the sternum.
- Note the respiratory rate and if breathing is normal or not.
- Listen to the heart and lungs.
- You should of course examine the abdomen, but in gastroenteritis, you should not expect to find anything significantly abnormal. Occasionally there is epigastric tenderness or other superficial (muscular) tenderness.

Examine the throat and ears, as viral infections often cause gastroenteritis and upper respiratory tract infection (URTI) at the same time.

In babies, look at the nappy area for rashes, which can be severe when there is diarrhoea.

If you happen to have a previous weight from within the past few weeks available, then it is useful to compare a re-weighing with this. Any drop in weight is mostly due to dehydration. If you work in an emergency department, make sure any child is weighed so that if they go home, this information will be available should the child come back.

Essentially, you are looking to reassure yourself that the child that you have examined is well and not significantly dehydrated or shocked. It is important to understand the difference between shock and dehydration when assessing children who have diarrhoea and vomiting. Although there is a relationship between these two physiologically abnormal states, they are different and should be managed differently.

Dehydration is the state of having a deficit of water compared to that needed for a healthy metabolism. **It takes at least hours and often days to become significantly dehydrated.** If more water is leaving the body than coming in, then the body will slowly transfer fluid from inside cells to keep the circulation well supplied. Dehydration is the state that occurs most commonly in children with diarrhoea and vomiting because it is an illness which undermines the body's ability to obtain fluid or hold onto fluid. The signs of dehydration are more to do with appearance than circulation and include dry mucous membranes, reduced skin turgor and sunken eyes. Dry mucous membranes usually appear first. When sunken eyes appear, dehydration is usually more advanced.

Shock or, more correctly in this context, hypovolaemia, is the state of having insufficient circulating volume to adequately perfuse all the tissues. The circulation is compromised, leading to a fast heart rate, delayed capillary refill and eventually low blood pressure. **If a child with diarrhoea and vomiting has signs of shock. it is for one of two reasons, neither of which are good news.** Either the dehydration is so severe or occurring so rapidly that the child cannot compensate and fails to maintain a good circulation, or the cause of the gastroenteritis is releasing toxins which have caused a state of septic shock, which have reduced the body's ability to maintain good tone in the blood vessels. In either case, **signs of shock indicate a medical emergency**.

 The 'must do's

- ☑ Any child who is sent home must be discharged with advice to return if they deteriorate.
- ☑ **Any child who is floppy or has an altered consciousness must have a blood sugar level checked.** Children with gastroenteritis use up their sugar reserves quickly and are not replacing them, so they are particularly prone to hypoglycaemia. Hypoglycaemia must be treated with oral glucose of some description in a child who is able to swallow, or intravenous 10% dextrose (5ml/kg bolus) in an unconscious child.

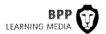

☑ In a general practice setting, buccal glucose gel is a reasonable temporary treatment for the collapsed child with hypoglycaemia.

Pitfalls to avoid

☒ The most common answer given by parents to questions about fluid intake and urine output is that both are completely absent. Frequently a flat response will be made by a parent despite a well looking child. Usually (but not always) the child is in fact drinking and urinating. The reason why the parent has told you that they are not doing so is because they do not want you to use a positive answer to dismiss their anxieties. The real answer would be 'yes, but not as much as usual'; however, because the parent subconsciously needs you to take their child's illness seriously, the answer becomes 'no'. Because you are a good and caring doctor, you will take the parents seriously but you also need to know what is really going on. The only way to achieve this is to ask the right questions and allow no room for interpretation. The questions that get a more realistic response are: 'When did your child last have a pee, even if it was only a little one?' (and) 'When did your child last have a bit to drink, even if they were sick soon afterwards?' Try these and see if you start to get different answers.

☒ **Intravenous therapy should only be started by a doctor who is experienced in prescribing fluids for children.** It would be very poor practice on any child to attach a bag of fluid to a cannula and 'run it through' without calculating an appropriate rate. Children can die from inappropriate fluid type or volume.

A guide to the management of diarrhoea and/or vomiting

If not dehydrated or significantly unwell:

If a child has diarrhoea or vomiting or both, and yet they are not significantly unwell with it, the best place for them is usually at home. Identify the reason for presenting so that you can address any concerns. Often there is an expectation that can be easily dealt with, such as 'We were told it was just a twenty-four hour bug Doc, but it's gone on for two days.' Often such illnesses can pass remarkably quickly, which is why the term exists. However, viral gastroenteritis affects everyone differently, even when they have the exact same infection and the length of illness can be extremely variable. Ultimately you can only assess that child at that moment in time. Persistence of symptoms in itself is not a reason to admit a child, though be aware that the more slowly dehydration develops, the more difficult it is to spot. Also, if symptoms continue without improvement for more than a few days, other causes become more likely.

Any child who appears well at the time of assessment can return later severely unwell. As a result, it is vital to have given good advice and offered an open door rather than an impression you are saying that 'there is nothing wrong' or 'it's only a viral tummy bug'. Useful advice includes:

- Offer the child to drink sips often. Drinking too much at once can make vomiting more likely.
- Give clear fluids, such as diluted juice and water. Something with a bit of sugar is ideal.
- Rehydration salts do get absorbed more quickly and so are very helpful, but they do taste funny and many children will not drink them. They are worth trying but the best rehydration fluid is the one which the child will drink, no matter what that is.

- Do not let any vomiting put you off giving drinks or medicines. You don't know how much stays down but it is usually more than you think.
- Expect the child to be not quite their normal selves but still alert and not floppy.
- Do not expect the child to eat at all. If they want to eat, avoid fatty, rich or spicy foods. Toast with jam but not butter is a good example of a good food for poorly tummies. Crisps and chocolates often make things worse.
- Tummy bugs are usually very bad for only two or three days. Usually the vomiting settles most quickly but the diarrhoea can take many days to go. The best way to judge the situation is by whether things are slowly improving.
- If at any point the child becomes floppy, drowsy (unless it is time for a sleep and they seem ok), stops drinking or stops urinating, they need to be seen again.
- If the diarrhoea is still significant in ten or so days, it could be that the tummy bug has affected the gut's ability to absorb milk. The child should cut all milk products out of the diet for a couple of weeks to see if that fixes things. If not then they should see their GP about the problem.

If mildly dehydrated or mildly unwell:

Because children do compensate well, and usually take hours at least to become seriously ill when they do so, it is safe to approach the child with some signs of illness or dehydration with a view to managing them without necessarily admitting them to hospital. **Often, children are seen at their worst just before they turn a corner**, and so if a change in tactic is made which improves matters then admission can be avoided.

Avoidance of intravenous fluid rehydration in children with gastroenteritis is desirable unless it is clearly needed. IV fluids should not be started on the premise that they are harmless. This is not the case. Although life-saving when given appropriately and with due care, any intravenous fluid therapy has affects on electrolyte and fluid balance that override the body's own regulation. As a result, intravenous rehydration has been associated with deaths due to brain oedema or low sodium. Where oral rehydration will be suitable, this is always preferable because giving fluids and salts enterally allows the body to regulate its intake and electrolyte levels.

Oral rehydration therapy can be given at home or in the emergency department depending on the wellness of the child and the resources available. In either circumstance, the aim is to maximise fluid intake and ensure that a child is reviewed if they fail to improve. There are various ways of getting children to drink when they have not done so thus far:

- **Offering fluids.** Sometimes fluids are not being offered at all at home. There is a myth that exists which says that by 'starving' a child of food and drink, the tummy bug will get better. This is completely untrue. Even children who are given nothing will continue to have diarrhoea and sometimes even vomiting.
- **Offering fluids every few minutes.** Large volumes are likely to make a child prone to vomiting and they do feel thirsty which makes them want to gulp. Some children are feeling so fed up that they just cannot be bothered to drink, which worsens the downward spiral of dehydration and lethargy. If these children are given a manageable sip every five minutes then this turns a downward spiral into an upwards trend.
- **Using a different way of giving fluids.** Try anything! Cups, beakers, bottles or syringes. If it works, go with it.
- **Using a different fluid.** Sometimes, babies have their milk confiscated for fear that it will make vomiting worse. This is another myth. Milk certainly makes vomitus offensive and can occasionally cause prolonged diarrhoea due to lactose intolerance. However as doctors we must avoid giving the impression

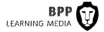

that children cannot have milk during gastroenteritis. Milk contains sugar and salt, both of which are needed and, for babies, it may be the only thing that they drink. Ultimately **the fluid which the child takes most readily is the best rehydration fluid**. Purpose-made rehydration salts do work well, however they taste salty and so children will often refuse them completely. A good alternative is diluted fruit cordial (avoid sugar free-cordials). Children with diarrhoea and vomiting need calories, and sweeteners are also laxatives.

- **Giving analgesia**. No-one really knows how children with gastroenteritis feel but I think that they feel pretty poorly. Viral illnesses give you aches and fevers, while vomiting and diarrhoea can both cause abdominal pain. Pain and general malaise both discourage drinking, thus contributing to the vicious cycle leading to dehydration. Medicines such as paracetamol are often not given to these children for fear of making the vomiting worse and out of a sense of fatalism that the dose will end up on the floor immediately afterwards. However, on the grounds that even if a child vomits, some of the dose may be retained, I use paracetamol to help turn these children around regularly. The effect is often dramatic. After about 30 to 60 minutes, a child who was disinterested starts to drink enthusiastically.

Any of these strategies can be used equally in hospital or trialled at home with suitable patients and sensible parents. After the attempt to improve fluid intake, there should be an improvement in the child. In my experience, parents are excellent judges of what constitutes a move in the right direction and should be encouraged to trust their instincts.

A child who fails to improve despite all of the above, or indeed worsens, should of course be referred to the paediatricians for further assessment.

If moderately dehydrated or moderately unwell:

Refer the following patients to the paediatric medical team:

- If a child has become **too unwell to be interested in drinking,** despite trying the previous measures.
- If a child has signs of **moderate dehydration** such as sunken eyes, poor urine output or 5% documented weight loss and poor fluid intake.
- If the **parents seem unable to cope** or the home circumstances are not satisfactory.
- If a child has any **signs of shock** such as tachycardia (not just raised heart rate during a fever), capillary refill of more than two seconds, floppiness or drowsiness (as opposed to tiredness), then they need urgent assessment. In addition to referral consider the following:
  - Fluid resuscitation is now likely to have to be intravenous and is best started sooner than later. If there is going to be a delay in the patient being seen and you are working somewhere with the right facilities, starting fluids with the right advice about the type and rate may make a big difference to the child's recovery.
  - Any child who seems significantly unwell with gastroenteritis should have a capillary blood glucose measured as soon as possible.

How to be a know-it-all

Not all diarrhoea and/or vomiting is actually viral gastroenteritis. As discussed in Chapter 6, appendicitis and viral gastroenteritis are sometimes confused. Other medical conditions such as inflammatory bowel disorders and other malabsorptions will present with diarrhoea, though vomiting is less commonly present and the onset is more insidious.

It is very difficult to reconcile that vomiting and diarrhoea at any age (but particularly in babies)

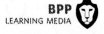

may be due to a urinary tract infection. When you couple this undeniable possibility with the fact that obtaining a sterile urine specimen from a child with diarrhoea is more that a bit of a challenge, you have a really unfair situation.

With this dilemma you can and probably will be caught out either way. If you never test urines when children have diarrhoea, you will miss urinary tract infections (UTI). If you test too many, you and your colleagues will have a never-ending supply of urine results which need repeating because there is something in there, but it's not clear if the specimen was contaminated. Completely clear urine specimens from a child with gastroenteritis are a rare gift.

In the context of general practice and emergency medicine, I think that it would be impractical to screen all children with vomiting and diarrhoea for urinary tract infection. However, the possibility should be considered, and I would suggest that **the following children should have a urine specimen tested one way or another:**

- Babies under six months old
- Any child who has vomiting but little or no diarrhoea
- Any child with a past history of UTI
- Any child who does not have a pattern of illness consistent with gastroenteritis, eg vomiting is persisting too long, no contact with other cases of diarrhoea and vomiting
- By being selective, it is possible to reduce the likelihood that you will miss a urinary tract infection that is pretending to be a viral gastroenteritis, without creating unnecessary stress for yourself, the children and the parents.

De-mystifying the role of the paediatrician: what the paediatrician might do

Often children with diarrhoea and vomiting will take an unexpected turn for the better, in which case they may be observed or allowed home. It is also possible that another tactic may be tried to achieve oral rehydration, or that nasogastric feeding will be tried. Practices vary widely with regard to preferences for oral, nasogastric and intravenous rehydration. Because of these possibilities, it is useful if referring doctors tell parents that the child is being referred for further assessment, rather than 'because they need a drip'.

 FAQs

Is it beneficial to give oral or nasogastric fluids to a child who is vomiting?

It is still quite common to see children present with vomiting and diarrhoea who are not receiving any oral fluids. This seems to be based on a belief that giving oral fluids will make vomiting worse. Both experience and evidence suggest that giving quite large amounts of enteral fluids to a vomiting child seems to be beneficial. What is certainly true is that restricting the intake of a vomiting child is a strategy which has no good basis.

Generally, enteral rehydration is preferable so that the child can better manage their own fluid and electrolyte balance. There are many strategies listed above that will improve the likelihood that enteral fluids will be successful. If after an initial assessment or failure of enteral rehydration, it is felt that this is not the best tactic for a particular child, then intravenous fluids should be prescribed by a clinician who has a good understanding of what to use and how much to give.

How long does this child need to stay off school?

Viral gastroenteritis is highly infectious. The likelihood is that most other children who are in an enclosed space with a child who vomits will develop some degree of infection themselves. Every year, entire schools and sometimes hospital wards have to close due to outbreaks

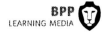

of what has been dubbed 'winter vomiting virus'. Transmission may well have already have taken place by the time you see the child since they have often been to school or nursery before anyone realised that they are unwell. To minimise further spread of infection it is essential that the child stays off school until the illness is over. Even after the child seems better, a period of 48 hours away from school is advised. This is partly because it is possible that the child may shed the virus after the infection is no longer clinically obvious, partly because children have relatively poor hand hygiene and also because infections can sometimes seem to resolve and then mysteriously start all over again.

When should I test a stool sample?

Stool microscopy and culture is usually unhelpful in children, since in the majority of cases the child will be well by the time a result is obtained. Generally speaking, a stool sample is more likely to be useful in the following circumstances:

- If the child has blood in the stools
- If the symptoms started during or after foreign travel
- For the more severely unwell children, especially if they require hospital admission
- Whenever a child is immunocompromised

What do I tell the parents?

When a child has gastroenteritis but is well enough to be managed at home:

"The most likely cause of your child's vomiting and diarrhoea is gastroenteritis, which is what we call a viral tummy infection. These infections are very common and most children will have a few tummy bugs as they grow up. Fortunately children have an incredible ability to cope with these illnesses. Although children can have quite a lot of vomiting and diarrhoea it is very rare for them to come to any harm."

"The only reason for being in hospital when a child has a tummy infection is if they need fluid through a drip. Having fluid through a drip requires a needle and there are some small risks to do with making sure the salt levels in the blood are safe. For this reason we only ever use drips to rehydrate children if we really need to, which is fortunately not often. The best way to get fluids into a child is to give them sips of clear fluids as often as possible."

"I think that at the moment, although your child is ill they do not need a drip, and so the best thing is to keep giving them sips of fluids to drink. This can be water, diluted cordial or fruit juice, or those drinks made from sachets which are made for people with diarrhoea. Most children who do this will get better. Even if they continue to vomit, children will usually absorb some of the liquid which they have drunk first. It is important to keep them drinking in between vomits. Do not worry about the fact that your child is not eating. This is because their tummy is sore. They will cope for now without any food and then make up for this when they are better."

"I can tell that your child is not too dry and dehydrated because they have a wet mouth, they have enough energy and they are still peeing. Occasionally children do get worse rather than better so you need to know what to look out for. It is best to come back to be seen again if your child becomes very drowsy in an unusual way, if they are too floppy, if they are completely refusing to drink or if you can just tell that they are getting worse. One of the best ways to tell if a child is not getting enough fluids is if they are not peeing enough. I think that while they are ill they might pee half as much as usual. If they are not even peeing this much or the pee is becoming brown instead of yellow, you should get your child seen again."

"I can't tell you exactly how soon your child will be better. This sometimes takes a few days. As long as your child is slowly getting better you should allow the infection to clear itself. If it reaches a point where it is not getting better from day to day then it may be useful to get your child reassessed."

Flowchart for assessing the child with diarrhoea and/or vomiting

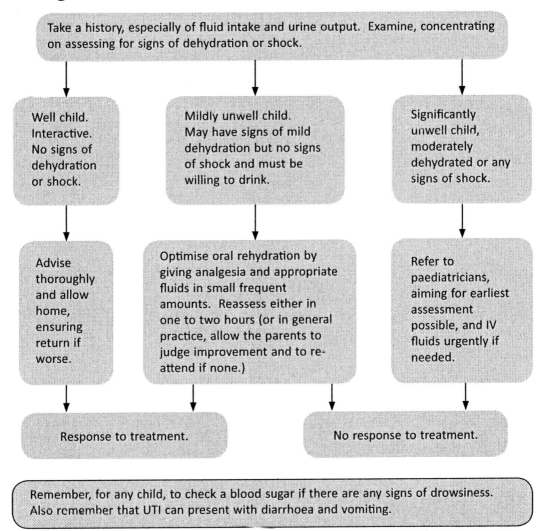

Take a history, especially of fluid intake and urine output. Examine, concentrating on assessing for signs of dehydration or shock.

Well child. Interactive. No signs of dehydration or shock.

Mildly unwell child. May have signs of mild dehydration but no signs of shock and must be willing to drink.

Significantly unwell child, moderately dehydrated or any signs of shock.

Advise thoroughly and allow home, ensuring return if worse.

Optimise oral rehydration by giving analgesia and appropriate fluids in small frequent amounts. Reassess either in one to two hours (or in general practice, allow the parents to judge improvement and to re-attend if none.)

Refer to paediatricians, aiming for earliest assessment possible, and IV fluids urgently if needed.

Response to treatment.

No response to treatment.

Remember, for any child, to check a blood sugar if there are any signs of drowsiness. Also remember that UTI can present with diarrhoea and vomiting.

Figure 9.1 Flowchart for assessing the child with diarrhoea and/or vomiting

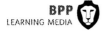

Summary for diarrhoea and/or vomiting

- Viral gastroenteritis is the cause of the majority of childhood vomiting and diarrhoea.
- Most cases are not brought to see a doctor, and of those that are, most need no specific medical intervention.
- Serious and life-threatening illness as a result of gastroenteritis is rare in the UK but does occur.
- Prevention of severe dehydration is best achieved by managing cases well at the stage where they can manage oral rehydration.
- It is preferable to increase enteral fluid intake than to withhold fluids.
- Treatment of severe dehydration is best managed by early recognition and careful but adequate intravenous rehydration.

Chapter 10

Non-accidental injury (NAI) and Child Protection concerns

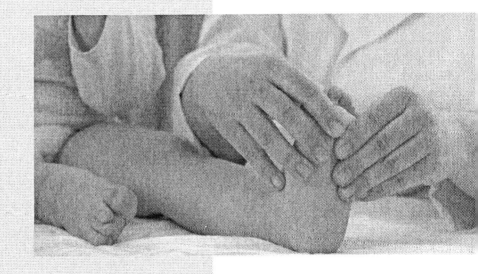

Non-accidental injury (NAI) and Child Protection concerns

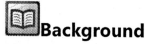

Background

If you are wondering why I have included this chapter, then I urge you to read on. Of course, I also urge you to read on if you weren't wondering that. **Child abuse is very common and takes many forms.** It can present in obvious ways but more frequently it is something that we will only pick up on if we have a constant awareness and vigilance. Its prevalence is difficult to assess due to its nature, but studies have put the prevalence in this country of sexual abuse alone as high as 11%, which is greater than the prevalence of asthma.

You have to be aware of the barriers to detecting any non-accidental harm to children and be mindful that the obstacles to uncovering abuse are multiple. You do not want to 'accuse' parents and this is because you value your relationship with them. You also have to acknowledge that when you assess children, you do so with a clinical eye. That is what makes you a good doctor. You focus on illness and sometimes this is at the cost of missing the social element of the child that you assess. By keeping your antennae up for possible child abuse, you will be an even better doctor.

This is probably the most difficult area of practice for any doctor who has contact with children, including paediatricians. However, it is important to have the courage to raise the issue and the majority of parents will not be offended if you explain the reasons for doing so. This is one area of paediatrics where fear of a thing is much worse than the thing itself. By being more confident when dealing with child protection matters, you will immediately find ourselves dealing with it more comfortably and efficiently.

How to assess

- Consider the possibility that abuse may be a factor in every encounter with children. **If you don't think about it you can't detect it.**
- Ask for details regarding anything that concerns you. Go into depth about the history.
- **Be specific about how injuries have happened.**
- If the child can communicate, be sure to ask them what happened before you ask the adults.
- Ask about the exact time, place and way that an injury occurred.
- Always **ask yourself, does this story fit what I am seeing?**
- Ask about the social circumstances.
- Ask whether there has been previous social services involvement and why.
- Ask about other children or siblings living in the home – have they ever had social services input?
- **Consider whether the parents/carers have acted appropriately.** Were they late in seeking medical attention? Could they have contributed to injury or ill health through inappropriate parenting?

The 'must do's

☑ **Consider NAI when seeing a child who attends multiple times for any reason.** In the high profile cases of recent years, the children who subsequently died of abuse often presented to medical professionals on many occasions with what was potentially identifiable NAI.

☑ **Document everything very clearly.**

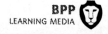

☑ **Examine the whole child** – you may find signs of neglect or of other injuries.

☑ **Discuss what you are doing with the parents/carers.** They need to know so that they understand what is happening. If you don't, they will find out eventually, and that will anger them far more than any perceived accusation.

☑ **Share your concerns** with someone. When you reach a level of concern where you are uncertain, then tell the carers this and make a phone call. Discuss the situation with the duty social worker, the trust's safeguarding children's nurse or on-call paediatric registrar. You can then agree on how to proceed.

☑ When contacting social workers, give them as much information as possible: current address and how long the family have lived there, names and dates of birth of all household members and significant contacts.

Pitfalls to avoid

☒ **Don't forget to keep the child's health as the priority.** For example, don't forget to give a child with a burn some pain relief, as well as dealing with child protection concerns.

☒ **Don't think of yourself as passing judgement.** No professional can take that responsibility. You have a duty to share concerns but something will only come of those concerns if other professionals add weight to your initial assessment. Think of it a bit like referring a child with abdominal pain and tenderness in the right iliac fossa. You haven't decided to take their appendix out but you wouldn't dream of sending them home, despite the fact that you know that from time to time, healthy appendices are removed. So you refer for a further assessment by someone who does take out appendices.

☒ If you are thinking to yourself 'I don't want to because…' then you are probably missing an opportunity to detect NAI.

☒ **Never refer without telling the parents that this is what you are doing.** If you do this and the parents choose not to go through with your referral, then they could legitimately say that they didn't see the need. If you have told them about your concerns and they still don't comply with any assessments, then you really are concerned now, aren't you?

☒ Never think 'these are such nice people and so they couldn't have neglected/ abused their child.' Experience shows us that abuse is sadly more easily concealed in families that give an outward appearance of 'normality'.

☒ Don't hold back for fear of consequences for the child. Despite reputations to the contrary, the professionals who do child protection work want to support families and only consider removing a child if the balance of risks justifies doing so.

☒ **Don't expect an abused child to be miserable.** They may be apparently normal or inappropriately friendly. They may be naughty or they may be subdued.

☒ Never half-document injuries. A lawyer may use this at a later date to claim that the injuries which you did not log either occurred after you saw them or were inconsistent and unreliably documented. The worst thing that could happen is that one inaccurate account of an injury undermines someone else's accurate description.

A guide to the management of NAI and Child Protection concerns

As a clinician who assesses children, it is extremely important that you should have a good idea of how to proceed when you or a

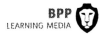

colleague has a child protection concern. The action that you take will depend greatly on the situation and the degree of concern.

In a general practice setting you may know the family from previous contacts and this can be both a help and a hindrance. It is important to recognise that because GPs tend to highly value the patient-doctor relationship, fear of damaging that relationship can be a barrier to considering and raising child protection concerns. On the other hand, as a family doctor you are in an excellent position to make an assessment. You can review the notes of other family members, discuss your concerns with other members of the team (practice nurse, receptionist, health visitor, school nurse, social worker, etc) and even visit the family home. You will also have a feel for what is appropriate health seeking behaviour and should listen to your gut feeling when something seems wrong.

In the emergency department or an acute assessment unit, there is still a desire to maintain good relationships with all patients and relatives or carers. There are additional resources that you can turn to more easily such as safeguarding nurses or consultants.

With regards to level of concern, I would suggest that it is useful to think of each case coming into one of three categories.

1. **There are cases where the situation caused you to consider NAI but after consideration you feel that this is very unlikely.** One example of this could be a head injury in a three-year-old which was witnessed by a third party whom you have spoken to. In these cases it is important to document your opinion and its basis. This is essential for two reasons. Firstly, should the child become a victim of abuse at a later date someone will look back at this episode and ask why you did not consider NAI. Secondly, if the child has further accidental injuries and a diligent doctor looks back on previous entries, it is

difficult for them to be reassured that any previous injuries were accidental unless someone has dutifully recorded that the possibility of NAI was considered.

2. **There are cases where you are neither convincingly concerned but nor are you reassured that NAI is satisfactorily excluded.** An example of this would be a delayed presentation of an injury but with no concerns about the injury's mechanism or about the child otherwise. Cases with low levels of concern are often the most difficult to handle. Realistically most will not be true NAIs, however, that does not mean that you should not take these cases further. While you may have reservations about raising the issue of safeguarding children in such cases, please consider the benefits of doing so even when no harm has been intended to the child:
   a. Every time you discuss safeguarding children, it reinforces the message to children, parents and carers that we consider child protection to be a serious issue. This might help a child to speak up one day either for themselves or someone else. It might even help someone to change their behaviour towards a child.
   b. Each case is an opportunity to improve safety or circumstances for the child even if no harm has been intended.
   c. The more that you get used to discussing child protection issues the better you will become at it. Like everything else in medicine, managing safeguarding issues is something that you will only do well if you take every opportunity to get involved.

So in these cases the best management is information-gathering and sharing. If you are uncertain about whether to refer a case you initially have two options. You can discuss the case with someone (an experienced colleague, a social worker, a safeguarding children's nurse or a paediatrician). Between you a decision can then be made regarding the next step. If you don't feel that you have

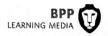

enough information to discuss the case, then you need to gather information from every source necessary until you are able to do so. Having discussed the case you may find that no further action is needed. You then need to document what was discussed and with whom.

Alternatively, following discussion you may agree that there is a significant ongoing concern. You can then discuss who will take that concern forward. Every locality should have a pathway in place for proceeding with child protection concerns. At some point during the process it is important to advise the child and carer what you are doing and why.

3. **There are the cases of presumed NAI.** In many ways these are more straightforward than the more uncertain second category. In these cases it is reasonable to refer early on, again following the local pathways that are in place. If it will not alter your decision to proceed, then it may be unnecessary duplication to gather too much background information. What is important is good documentation, good delivery of the information which you have to the people who will take the case forward. and openness with the parents and child.

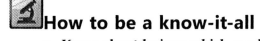

How to be a know-it-all

- **Know about lesions which can look like injuries.** The two most common are:
  - Mongolian blue spots pretending to be bruises, and;
  - Bullous impetigo pretending to be a scald.
- Consider conducting some checks of your own – call the health visitor, school nurse, GP, previous GP or anyone who might be able to give further information. You may find that others also have niggling doubts and

concerns and that you are the first to do something for this child.

Also worth knowing

- The degree of certainty needed for child protection is based on the 'balance of probabilities'. This is different from criminal law where the court has to be convinced 'beyond reasonable doubt'. This, of course, is the threshold for deciding whether abuse has taken place. The threshold for concern should be much lower, and may include cases where neglect, harm, emotional or physical abuse is at a significant risk of occurring.

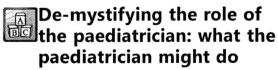

De-mystifying the role of the paediatrician: what the paediatrician might do

Paediatricians are available to advise and assess where appropriate. They may not be the most appropriate person to approach initially and most referrals will go through social care services before involving a children's doctor. The most common reason for involving a doctor in child protection cases is to document lesions, give an opinion as to their likely origin and put this information in the context of the social background.

Where medical input is needed, a thorough child protection assessment needs to be performed by someone with the appropriate training and who does this work regularly.

The paediatrician will:

- Obtain the important background information from health and social care workers, in order to understand the circumstances and degree of concern that exists for any people involved.

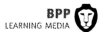

- Take a careful history from anyone involved. It is difficult to determine whether injuries fit a story unless you have the full story.
- Examine the child fully, including a full (staged) exposure of the child's skin. The child should also be weighed, measured and plotted on a growth chart.
- Draw diagrams of and possibly photograph anything found.
- Possibly arrange for blood tests, X-rays and scans to further assess.
- Discuss their assessment with social workers and the appropriate members of the child's family (or child's carers).

It is then the role of the social care team to decide regarding action. This will range from deciding that they are satisfied that no abuse is likely to a high level of concern. The immediate outcome will then depend on the circumstances.

FAQs

Is vaginal discharge suspicious of abuse?

This question raises many of the issues that make detecting child abuse so difficult. Injuries can happen accidentally but they should make us consider NAI. Vaginal discharge may be medical or physiological. Most vaginal discharges are unrelated to abuse, however, they are more common in abused children. The important thing is to consider the possibility of abuse. Similarly, anal fissures may be due to constipation but it would be awful if in a particular child's case the anal trauma was due to abuse and no one dared to think that this was the case.

In particular, it is worth considering that outside of puberty, and the period when children are in nappies, thrush is less common. Poor hygiene or over-zealous cleaning of genitals can both cause vaginal discharge at any age. I would recommend, that if you are initially reassured in these children that you do not otherwise suspect abuse, then give toileting advice (wipe front to back with a fresh sheet of toilet paper each time after passing stools, until you get two clean wipes) and bathing advice (wash your privates with water only and don't use bubble bath) and arrange for a review in 2–4 weeks. If the discharge persists, I would suggest referral to a general paediatrician at this point.

For pubertal girls, before deciding that a discharge is physiological, make every effort to talk to the young person alone. If they are sexually active, whether consensual or not, anyone who cares for that child will be grateful that you do so.

I raise the issue of abuse in all children who present with anal fissures or vaginal discharge, but do so in a way that makes it clear that this it is part of my job to always ask. Initially I prefer to simply ask the accompanying adult whether they or anyone else have ever had concerns that someone may be abusing their child. One of the principles of child protection is that while you might only do a detailed investigation when you have reason to do so, it is better to ask than avoid discussing the issue of abuse for fear of causing offence.

How can I tell a non-accidental bruise from an accidental bruise?

You can't often say that any particular finding is due or not due to abuse. What you should be doing is deciding whether you are convinced that NAI is very unlikely in any given circumstance. If we allow ourselves to fall into the trap of waiting until we are very concerned, then we will detect abuse too late. Remember that you are not making a judgement but rather trying to protect all children by acting when appropriate. Unfortunately, this does mean inconveniencing both parents and ourselves, because it is necessary to have a low threshold for in-depth assessment where NAI is a significant possibility.

So in order to determine what should concern you, consider the following:

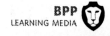

Factors which make abuse more likely:

- Injuries in a child who is not yet mobile.
- Injuries which do not fit the history given.
- Injuries in areas which do not usually happen by accident eg on the back, on the neck or on the pinna.
- Previous abuse.
- Delay in presentation.
- Other children in the family/home who have been assessed and who became subject to a child protection plan (or were 'on the child protection register' as it used to be termed).

Factors which make abuse less likely:

- A clear history which fits the injury and is plausible.
- A history given freely by the child, who gives further plausible detail when asked.
- Injuries that are in areas which are commonly prone to knocks, eg shins.

Some injuries do look suspicious. One example is small circular burns, which should make you think of cigarette burns. Sometimes linear bruises can indicate slap marks. However, it is possible to be fooled either way. The important thing is to get enough information to make a good decision.

Note that all trusts will have very detailed protocols in place for managing safeguarding children. The following flowcharts provide an overview of how to approach safeguarding issues.

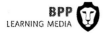

Flowchart for assessing suspected physical abuse

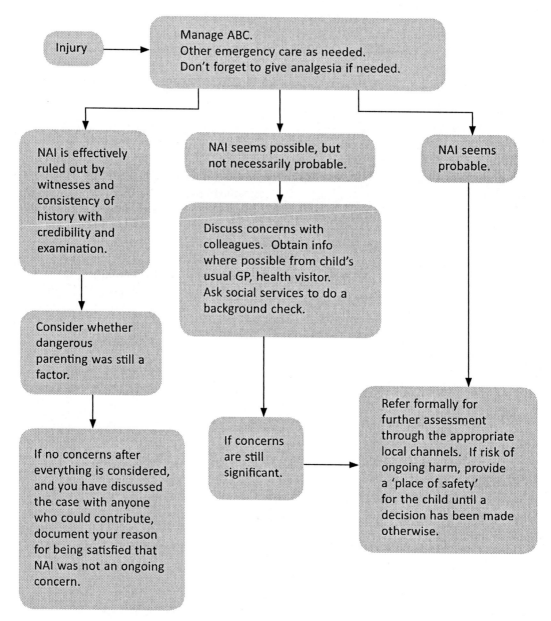

Figure 10.1 Flowchart for assessing suspected physical abuse

Flowchart for assessing suspected physical neglect or emotional abuse

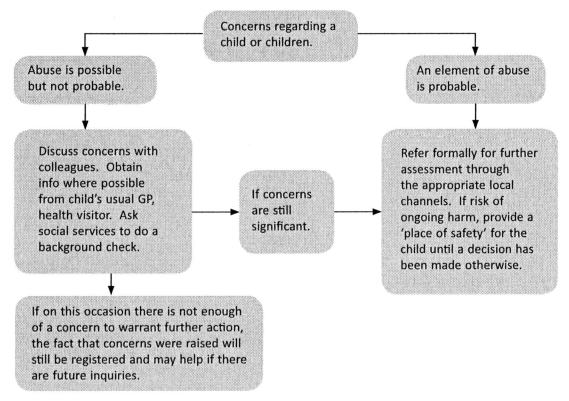

Figure 10.2 Flowchart for assessing suspected physical neglect or emotional abuse

Flowchart for assessing suspected sexual abuse

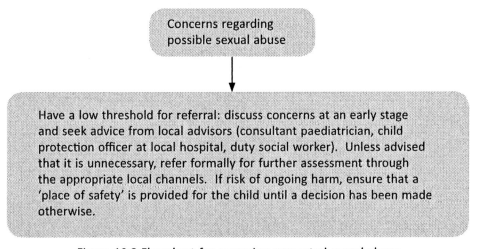

Figure 10.3 Flowchart for assessing suspected sexual abuse

What do I tell the parents?

Firstly, let me emphasise how important good communication is in dealing with child protection. It is all too easy to avoid the issue when in these circumstances. However, this will damage trust and leave you open to criticism. If, for example, a parent is told that their child 'just needs further assessment', then the person who failed to explain the importance of attending will be responsible when that parent fails to attend. After all, many parents do not bring their child to an outpatients appointment for various reasons. Also, should the parent come to the assessment as requested, they will be understandably aggrieved that they have been misled by not having the reasons for the said assessment explained.

So, I always start with honesty. **Explain what needs to happen, and why it is important.** Being the person to tell the parents that a child protection assessment is needed will create an understandable fear in anyone who is not used to doing this. The anxiety is that the parents/carers will feel accused, and that they will see you no longer as their doctor, but someone sitting in judgement over them. It really doesn't have to be like that though, and the way to avoid these reactions from parents is relatively straightforward:

1. Use the first person plural wherever possible. Don't say '*I* need to refer *your* child because *they* have some bruises which *you* cannot explain.' Instead explain that 'as doctors, we need to refer any child who has some bruises which cannot easily be explained.' By using this kind of language you tell it how it is. You haven't made a judgement, but rather decided to arrange an appropriate assessment. If your language reflects this, then parents and carers will respond better.

2. Explain the importance and put it in context. Most people are aware now of horrific child abuse cases which have been in the news. By explaining to parents that with their co-operation, we can help to prevent further cases, you will find the reasonable majority willing to cooperate.

3. Having explained the 'why', explain 'what will happen'. Be honest that people will need to ask a lot of seemingly unusual and often personal questions that the child will need to be thoroughly examined and that tests may be necessary.

When I need to refer for a child protection assessment or do one myself:

"Part of my job is to make sure that all children are safe. In order to do that, I have to make sure that whenever a child comes with something that isn't straightforward, I make sure that we fully explain what has happened. Sadly this is because some adults do hurt or neglect children. I am sure that you are aware of examples from the news."

"I realise that most parents/carers do not hurt their children but in order to make sure that we pick up on it when it does happen, we have to be very thorough. Your help in doing this is very important and also helps for any assessment to finish more quickly."

"It is important that you understand that in order to do this, we have to make sure that all the people involved such as GPs, health visitors and social workers communicate with each other and share information."

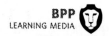

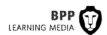 Summary for non-accidental injury (NAI) and Child Protection concerns

- Child abuse is common and often undetected even when at its worst.
- An open and honest approach helps to make child protection less confrontational.
- It is important to have an open mind and consider NAI in all contact with children, especially if there has been an injury.
- Even if there is only a low level of concern, it is worth discussing with a colleague.
- It is good to have a low threshold for discussion with social workers or safeguarding children team workers. Get to know your local referral and advisory pathways.

Closing Thoughts

I have written this book based on my experience in general practice and my career as a hospital paediatrician. I intend it to be a practical guide to common paediatric problems for anyone who assesses sick children whether in general practice, the emergency department or a general paediatric assessment unit. It is designed to reflect clinical presentations rather than physiological and anatomical systems, and for this reason it is divided into chapters which reflect presenting complaints.

Medicine is now becoming dominated by guidelines and protocols which are intended to support clinicians but can also restrict us. This book is meant to help you to develop your 'sixth sense' and I hope that using it will increase confidence and satisfaction when trying to make sense of children who present acutely. By having an idea of how to approach each mode of presentation, I hope that you will enjoy your time treating children more. This in turn will increase the trust that parents and children have in you. Also I anticipate that, just occasionally, you will enjoy a smug feeling which comes from being a bit of a know-it-all when dealing with sick children.

Paediatrics is the branch of medicine where you can still spend most of your clinical time treating illness and have fun doing so! As soon as you know what you are looking for, you can discover the best thing about paediatrics: there really is no science to most of it, so you get to use your clinical judgment! Sound exciting? Well, it is.

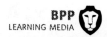

Index

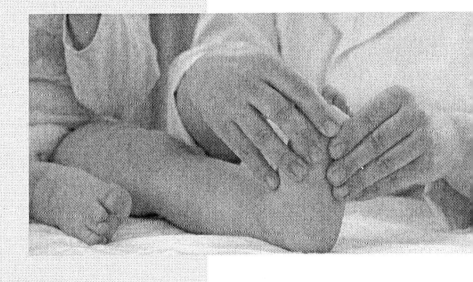

Index

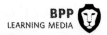

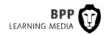

More titles in the Progressing your Medical Career Series

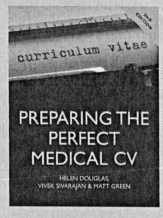

PREPARING THE PERFECT MEDICAL CV

HELEN DOUGLAS,
VIVEK SIVARAJAN & MATT GREEN

October 2011
Paperback
978-1-445381-62-6

Are you unsure of how to structure your Medical CV? Would you like to know how to ensure you stand out from the crowd?

With competition for medical posts at an all time high it is vital that your Medical CV stands out over your fellow applicants. This comprehensive, unique and easy-to-read guide has been written with this in mind to help prospective medical students, current medical students and doctors of all grades prepare a Medical CV of the highest quality. Whether you are applying to medical school, currently completing your medical degree or a doctor progressing through your career (foundation doctor, specialty trainee in general practice, surgery or medicine, GP career grade or Consultant) this guide includes specific guidance for applicants at every level.

This time-saving and detailed guide:

- Explains what selection panels are looking for when reviewing applications at all levels.

- Discusses how to structure your Medical CV to ensure you stand out for the right reasons.

- Explores what information to include (and not to include) in your CV.

- Covers what to consider when maintaining a portfolio at every step of your career, including, for revalidation and relicensing purposes.

- Provides examples of high quality CVs to illustrate the above.

This unique guide will show you how to prepare your CV for every step of your medical career from pre-Medical School right through to Consultant level and should be a constant companion to ensure you secure your first choice post every time.

BPP
LEARNING MEDIA

More titles in the Progressing your Medical Career Series

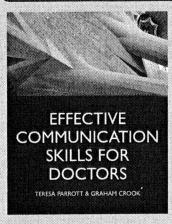

EFFECTIVE
COMMUNICATION
SKILLS FOR
DOCTORS

TERESA PARROTT & GRAHAM CROOK

September 2011
Paperback
978-1-445379-56-2

Would you like to know how to improve your communication skills? Are you looking for a clearly written book which explores all aspects of effective medical communication?

There is an urgent need to improve doctors' communication skills. Research has shown that poor communication can contribute to patient dissatisfaction, lack of compliance and increased medico-legal problems. Improved communication skills will impact positively on all of these areas.

The last fifteen years have seen unprecedented changes in medicine and the role of doctors. Effective communication skills are vital to these new roles. But communication is not just related to personality. Skills can be learned which can make your communication more effective, and help you to improve your relationships with patients, their families and fellow doctors.

This book shows how to learn those skills and outlines why we all need to communicate more effectively. Healthcare is increasingly a partnership. Change is happening at all levels, from government directives to patient expectations. Communication is a bridge between the wisdom of the past and the vision of the future.

Readers of this book can also gain free access to an online module which upon successful completion can download a certificate for their portfolio of learning/Revalidation/CPD records.

This easy-to-read guide will help medical students and doctors at all stages of their careers improve their communication within a hospital environment.

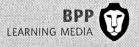

BPP
LEARNING MEDIA

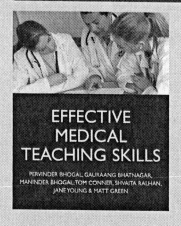
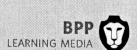

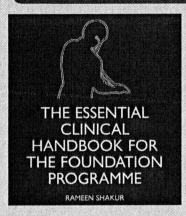
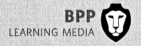

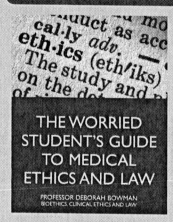
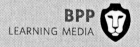